Endomorph Diet

Beginners Guide with 100 Recipes and 30 Day Meal Plan for Losing Weight and Staying Fit. Breakfast, Lunch, Dinner, Dessert Recipes

Author: Kate Princeton Johnson

Copyright 2020 by Kate Princeton Johnson - All rights reserved.

This document is geared towards providing exact and reliable information in regard to the topic and issue covered. The publication is sold on the idea that the publisher is not required to render an accounting, officially permitted, or otherwise, qualified services. If advice is necessary, legal or professional, a practiced individual in the profession should be ordered.

From a Declaration of Principles which was accepted and approved equally by a Committee of the American Bar Association and a Committee of Publishers and Associations.

In no way is it legal to reproduce, duplicate, or transmit any part of this document by either electronic means or in printed format. Recording of this publication is strictly prohibited and any storage of this document is not allowed unless with written permission from the publisher. All rights reserved.

The information provided herein is stated to be truthful and consistent, in that any liability, in terms of inattention or otherwise, by any usage or abuse of any policies, processes, or Directions: contained within is the solitary and utter responsibility of the recipient reader. Under no circumstances will any legal responsibility or blame be held against the publisher for any reparation, damages, or monetary loss due to the information herein, either directly or indirectly.

Readers acknowledge that the author is not engaging in the rendering of legal, financial, medical or professional advice.

By continuing with this book, readers agree that the author is under no circumstances responsible for any losses, indirect or direct, that are incurred as a result of the information presented in this document, including, but not limited to inaccuracies, omissions and errors

Respective authors own all copyrights not held by the publisher.

The information herein is offered for informational purposes solely and is universal as so. The presentation of the information is without a contract or any type of guarantee assurance.

The trademarks that are used are without any consent, and the publication of the trademark is without permission or backing by the trademark owner. All trademarks and brands within this book are for clarifying purposes only and are the owned by the owners themselves, not affiliated with this document.

Contents

- Introduction 8
- What is Endomorph Diet? Why it is important? 9
- How do you tell if you are an endomorph? 9
- Food Items to Eat on Endomorph Diet 11
- Polyunsaturated and Monounsaturated Fats 12
- Food to Avoid During Endomorph Diet 13
- Weight and Strength Training Exercises 15
- Breakfast Recipes 21
- Recipe 01: Chicken Salad Wrap 21
- Recipe 02: Scrambled Eggs with Spinach 22
- Recipe 03: Yummy Spinach Omelet 23
- Recipe 04: Savory Brownies 24
- Recipe 05: Vegan Muffin 25
- Recipe 06: Cauliflower Rice 26
- Recipe 07: Peach Smoothie 27
- Recipe 08: Green Smoothie 28
- Recipe 09: Pineapple Smoothie 29
- Recipe 10: Beetroot Smoothie 30
- Recipe 11: Kale Smoothie 31
- Recipe 12: Almond Chocolate Milk 32
- Recipe 13: Protein Berry Smoothie 33
- Recipe 14: Strawberry Smoothie 34
- Recipe 15: Blueberry Smoothie 35

Recipe 16: Yummy Quiche 36

Recipe 17: Egg Scrambled and Vegetables 37

Recipe 18: Yogurt Parfait 38

Recipe 19: Yogurt Pancakes 39

Recipe 20: Cheese Casserole 40

Recipe 21: Oatmeal Muffins 41

Recipe 22: Cinnamon and Apple Toast 42

Lunch Recipes 43

Recipe 23: Chicken Parmesan 43

Recipe 24: Mushroom Chicken 44

Recipe 25: Chicken Fajitas 45

Recipe 26: Mouthwatering Fish Burgers 46

Recipe 27: Tasty Parmesan Shrimps with Garlic 47

Recipe 28: Tuna Salad and Cranberry 48

Recipe 29: Summer Squash with Black Beans 49

Recipe 30: Chicken Pasta 50

Recipe 31: Spinach Manicotti 51

Recipe 32: Potato Soup 52

Recipe 33: Apricot BBQ Chicken 53

Recipe 34: Chicken Sautéed Rice 54

Recipe 35: Tasty Chili 55

Recipe 36: Yummy Chicken Fajita 56

Recipe 37: Baked Salmon 57

Recipe 38: Chicken Nuggets 58

Recipe 39: Chicken Verde 59

Recipe 40: Chickpea Salad 60

Recipe 41: Grilled Shrimps 61

Recipe 42: Cod Fillets 62

Recipe 43: Grilled Chicken 63

Recipe 44: Chinese Soup 64

Recipe 45: Baked Red Pepper 65

Recipe 46: Balsamic Bruschetta 66

Recipe 47: Guacamole 67

Recipe 48: Jalapeno Spread 68

Recipe 49: Avocado Salad 69

Recipe 50: Roasted Vegetables 70

Recipe 51: Butter Squash Noodles 71

Recipe 52: Fruity Chicken Salad 72

Recipe 53: Nutty Chicken Salad 73

Recipe 54: Black Beans Salad 74

Recipe 55: Ricotta Pie with Swiss Chard 75

Recipe 56: Yummy Pumpkin Bread 77

Recipe 57: Lunch Casserole 78

Recipe 58: Tofu Bites 79

Recipe 59: Vegetable Chili 80

Recipe 60: Bell Pepper 81

Recipe 61: Roasted Bell Pepper and Tofu 82

Dinner Recipes 83

Recipe 62: Roasted Turkey 83

Recipe 63: Roasted Pork 84

Recipe 64: Beef Bulgogi 85

Recipe 65: BBQ Ribs 86

Recipe 66: Roasted Lamb 87

Recipe 67: Fish Fillets 88

Recipe 68: Chickpea Salad 89

Recipe 69: Tortilla Chips 90

Recipe 70: Zucchini Chips 91

Recipe 71: Dinner Meatballs 92

Recipe 72: Salmon Cake 93

Recipe 73: Chicken with Coconut Milk 94

Recipe 74: Spinach Soup 95

Recipe 75: Beef Soup 96

Recipe 76: Gherkins Salad 97

Recipe 77: Shrimp Harissa 98

Recipe 78: Onion Soup 99

Dessert Recipes 100

Recipe 79: Apple Cake 100

Recipe 80: Diet Bites 101

Recipe 81: Sugar-free Pie 102

Recipe 82: Pumpkin Pie 103

Recipe 83: Almond Bars 104

Recipe 84: Apple Sorbet 105

Recipe 85: Choco Dates 106

Recipe 86: Macaroon 107

Recipe 87: Pancake 108

Appetizer Recipe 109

Recipe 88: Almond and Chicken Snack 109

Recipe 89: Salmon with Soya Beans 110

Recipe 90: Chicken Skewer 111

Recipe 91: Lentil Sandwich 113

Recipe 92: Cornflakes Cookies 114

Recipe 93: Coconut Cookies 115

Recipe 94: Chocolate Rice Bars 116

Recipe 95: Peanut Choco Bars 117

Recipe 96: Baked Marshmallow Treats 118

Recipe 97: Choco Log 119

Recipe 98: Crispy Rice Treats with Nuts 120

Recipe 99: Caramel Cheese Bars 121

Recipe 100: Brownie Bars 122

Conclusion 123

Introduction

Do you want to define your muscles while dropping extra pounds? Dietitians often recommend following a regular exercise routine and a healthy diet. You will need a diet plan based on the type of your body. Some workout plans may be better than others. Fortunately, you can get a plan according to the type of your body.

If your body has little muscles and a high percentage of fat, you have an endomorph body. Unfortunately, people with this type of body may struggle with their weight loss. It is crucial to understand how your body is different from several other types. Moreover, you have to find out what is good to consume and what is not suitable to eat.

Metabolism of the endomorph body type is slower than others. As a result, it will be easy for you to gain weight and difficult to shed extra pounds. It can also impact your muscle growth. Though, you can get the advantage of an endomorph diet plan to maintain and meet your health goals.

People with this type of body have round, soft bodies with large bones, hips, and joints. This book covers what an endomorph diet is, and the right foods to avoid and eat. Moreover, you will find out the best exercises and recipes to build muscle and lose weight. All these things are suitable for people with endomorph bodies.

I am going to share a comprehensive diet based on my research and personal experience. No doubt, people having an endomorphic body may have traits and characteristics that make it complicated for them to increase muscle mass, exercise, or diet.

Specialists have designed endomorph exercise plans and diets that work against these traits to help people lose weight. Bodies of these people have a slow metabolism because of their substantial build. A slow metabolism means that your body is prone to convert extra calories into fat.

For people having endomorphic bodies, it cannot be easy to follow exercise and diet plans. For instance, they generally have desires for comfort and food. These people carry extra weight and have a large body; therefore, they will be prone to sedentarism. Moreover, it is difficult for you to gain impressive muscle mass because extra body fat will trigger to release estrogen.

An increase in the level of estrogen may decrease testosterone. Remember, testosterone is an important hormone to promote the growth of muscles. No doubt, weight loss is a significant struggle for endomorphs. In this book, we are going to share essential exercises, food items, diet plans, and recipes for your assistance to achieve your fitness goal. If you enjoy reading this book, please leave your feedback. Your few words will help people to understand if this book is suitable for them to lose weight.

What is Endomorph Diet? Why it is important?

Before diving into the details of the endomorph diet, it is essential to explain the meaning of endomorph. Remember, it is a round body type with large bones. Two other body types are mesomorph and ectomorph. Mesomorphs are muscular and hourglass-shaped bodies. Meanwhile, ectomorphs are thin with skinny, long limbs.

A person with a large bone structure, large wrists and ankles is an endomorph. They can easily store fat and lack defined muscles. These types of bodies use sugar as a source of fuel; therefore, it is difficult to burn fat. Undoubtedly, they have a slow metabolism, but it can be easy for them to build muscles.

People with endomorph body often feel like gaining weight by looking at food. Your body may store fat even after eating less food. For this reason, having an endomorph body can be an actual struggle. Their slower metabolism will make it challenging to burn off calories from food. You should not take tension because the Endomorph diet is available for your assistance. Before using this diet, it is crucial to find out if you are an endomorph.

How do you tell if you are an endomorph?

Initially, it can be difficult to tell if you are an endomorph. If you are overweight, it does not mean that you are an endomorph. An endomorph might suffer from skinny fat syndrome. It is a condition in which a person has low muscle mass and higher body fat. As a result, your stomach will stick out.

You are an ectomorph if you have to drop extra body fat and add extra muscle mass to solve this problem. To evaluate your body type, wrap your middle finger and thumb around an opposing wrist. If your thumb and middle finger do not wrap around to touch each other, you are an endomorph.

In case, your middle finger and thumb wrap around perfectly to touch each other, you are a mesomorph. If your index finger and thumb overlap each other, you will be an ectomorph. Marilyn Monroe, Sophia Vergara, and Jennifer Lopez are some famous endomorphs. They have small-waist, pear-shape, full-figure, and curvaceous bodies.

They are famous for their round, smooth body, small shoulders, short limbs, and medium-large structure of bone. Their fat distribution pattern makes it difficult to lose weight. If you want to lose weight, you have to follow the correct nutrition and training program.

Metabolic Characteristics

People with endomorph body types have insulin and carbohydrate sensitivity. High-carb food items are immediately converted to sugar in your bloodstream. These may be stored as fat instead of burning for energy. The fat percentage can be high in several endomorphs. It can increase their risk of developing infertility, diabetes, cancer, heart disease, gallbladder conditions, depression, and hypertension. You can prevent hormone imbalance with a fitness and nutrition program to reduce body fat.

Weight Loss and Diet

Endomorphs are sensitive to insulin and carbohydrate. The best diet plan for this type of body focuses on the equal supply of macronutrients with carbohydrates from high-fiber, unrefined scratches (amaranth and quinoa) and vegetables. Avoid consumption of cookie, cracker, cereal, and bread aisles of a supermarket. Your meals should contain healthy fats, such as olive oil or avocado, vegetables, and protein. For your meals, you can consider 35% fat, 35% protein, and 30% carbs.

Food Items to Eat on Endomorph Diet

With an endomorphic body, you will need a particular fitness plan to shed pounds. The endomorphic fitness type is suitable for your body. As per the theory of this diet, endomorphs have a slow metabolism. You may not be able to burn calories like mesomorphs and ectomorphs. Extra calories can be converted into fats. Moreover, you do not have sufficient tolerance to carbohydrates.

The best diet for your body may have a high protein and fat intake. It may be similar to a paleo diet. Remember, the diet may help you to lose fat while improving the energy of your body. Some excellent sources of proteins and fats are:

- Olive oil
- Macadamia nuts
- Beef
- Fatty fish
- Egg yolk
- Walnuts
- Cheese

There is no need to avoid carbohydrates. Carbs offer sufficient energy to your body. By removing carbohydrates from your meals, you may feel fatigued and sluggish. Moreover, extremely low carbohydrates in your diet may increase the chances of gastrointestinal issues. For this reason, choose complex carbohydrates, such as vegetables. Starchy vegetables, such as tubers, potatoes, whole grains, fruits, and legumes are good sources of complex carbs.

You must not consume simple carbohydrates. These foods have high calories and sugar that may increase the chances of fat storage. Simple carbohydrates have white bread, cookies, cakes, pasta, and white rice.

The fruit is essential for the endomorph diet. If you are carb-sensitive, eat fruits in a moderate amount. In your meals, you can consider 35% fat, 35% protein, and 30% carbohydrates. Portion control plays an important role to decrease body fat. It will help you to decrease calorie consumption. Try to eat almost 200 – 500 less calories that you usually consume. In this way, you can shed pounds and reach a weight loss goal.

Polyunsaturated and Monounsaturated Fats

It is vital to consume food rich in healthful monounsaturated and polyunsaturated fats or protein. The list includes:

- Dairy (low fat) products, including cheeses, yogurt, and low-fat milk
- Poultry, including turkey and chicken
- Several nontropical vegetable oils, such as avocado oil, canola, and olive
- Different fish types, particularly fatty fish
- Egg whites and egg
- Nontropcial nuts, such as walnuts, hazelnuts, and almonds

Your body needs sufficient carbohydrates. Here are some good examples to fit in your endomorph diet:

- Fruits (avoid pineapple and melons)
- Legumes and dried beans, including chickpeas, lentils, and kidney beans
- Whole-wheat and whole-grain products, including whole-wheat bread and all-bran cereal
- Non-starchy veggies, including celery, cauliflower, and broccoli
- Starchy vegetables, including carrots, corn, yams, and sweet potatoes
- Unrefined starchy veggies, including amaranth and quinoa

Food to Avoid During Endomorph Diet

People with this type of body are sensitive to insulin and carbohydrates. Remember, insulin hormone helps blood sugars to move in cells. For an endomorph diet, you have to avoid or limit carbohydrate dense foods, including sugar and white flour.

Foods with carbohydrates can quickly release sugars in your bloodstream. As a result, you will notice dips and spikes in blood sugar. The body can turn sugars into fat instead of burning them to produce energy.

Endomorphic bodies can convert extra calories into fat. Therefore, people following this diet should avoid nutrient-poor and calorie-dense food. Some food items are prohibited in the endomorph diet, such as:

- Bagels, traditional pasta, white rice, and white bread
- Sweets, chocolates, and candies
- Cakes and baked goods
- Sports drinks, energy drinks, and soft drinks
- Refined cereals, including puffed rice, instant oatmeal, and bran flakes
- Fried or processed foods
- Dairy products, including ice cream, whipped cream, and cream
- Red meats
- Alcohol
- Cooking oils with saturated fat, including coconut or palm oil
- Food with sodium
- Endomorph Workout Plan

No doubt, endomorphs find it difficult to lose their body fat. For this reason, dieting alone may not help. You have to include physical activity in your regular routine. It is an important recommendation to improve your health.

A weight loss plan is incomplete without exercise, especially for the endomorph body type. Exercise allows you to reduce fat and increase metabolism. Cardiovascular exercises, including running, will help you to burn calories. You have to burn more calories than your consumption. Make sure to burn extra fat.

As per ACE (American Council on Exercise), people with this body type must follow a well-rounded exercise. You have to focus on strength training and cardiovascular activities. See these examples:

HIIT (High-Intensity Interval Training): In HIIT, you have to alternate between different periods of low intensity and high-intensity exercise along with rest. For your endomorphic body, HIIT sessions are suitable. You can do this exercise for 2 – 3 times per week. Each session must be 30 minutes long.

SST (Steady State Training): These may be long sessions of low to moderate-intensity exercise. Some suitable SST exercises are swimming, jogging, and walking. If you have an endomorph body type, you can follow SST for almost 30 to 60 minutes three times a week.

Weight and Strength Training Exercises

If you want to build muscles, you can follow strength training exercises. It must be an important part of your weight loss plan for people with an endomorph body. The muscle mass of these people will be low; however, they have wide, large bones capable of bearing strong and large muscles. They often have extra body fat that increases estrogen levels and decreases testosterone levels. As a result, you will notice a hindrance to muscle growth.

A healthy muscle group is necessary to increase metabolism because muscle tissues can burn calories. They help your body to use fat for fuel. Several exercises and weight training routines are useful for endomorphic bodies. Experts recommend several compound exercises. With the help of compound exercises, you can use different units and body tissues. It offers the best control of your body. You can use bodyweight, barbell, and free weights during exercise. Some compound exercises include:

Hip Hinge and Deadlift

You can do deadlifts or hip hinges to lose weight. Here are some simple instructions to do these exercises:

- Stand with legs hip-width at a distance and near the barbell.
- Drive your hips back when bracing the core and manage tension in the knee and back soft, and push your heels on the floor.
- Once the bar reaches the knees, you can shoot hips into a bar.
- When compressing the glutes, stand tall.

Pushups

- If you want to do pushups, here are some important instructions to follow.
- Put your hands on the floor, spread fingers widely and directly under your shoulders.
- Squeeze your glutes, pack your shoulders, and press your heels away.
- Keep your head in line with your body, bend elbows, and low down the chest toward the ground with proper control.
- Keep your head aligns with your body, bend elbows, and lower your chest toward the ground with absolute control.
- Keep your back straight while engaging glutes, shoulders, and legs to raise the chest again.

Squats

- Stand with your legs (shoulder-width) apart, drive your feet in the ground, and activate your hips.
- Slowly move your tailbone down toward the ground with an engaged and tall torso.
- Once lowered, push your body away slowly from the ground until standing with the fully extended torso.

Circuit Training

Expert recommends circuit training for people endomorph body types. This training comprises of intense, short bouts of exercises with some rest in-between. Here is an example of this training:

- Squat and overhead press for 50 seconds
- Rest for 10 seconds
- Stationary lunges with right leg front, lateral raise for 50 seconds
- Rest for 10 seconds
- Stationary lunge and lateral raise, hold dumbbells for left leg front (50 seconds)
- Rest for 10 seconds
- Upright row or plie squat, kettlebell or dumbbells for 50 seconds
- Rest for ten seconds
- Pushup for 50 seconds with knee drives the single leg
- Rest for 10 seconds
- Plank with dumbbells along with triceps extension for 50 seconds
- Rest for 10 seconds
- Substitute step-ups with dumbbells, hammer curls for 50 seconds
- Replicate all these steps for almost three times

Endomorph Diet Plan for 30 Days

Day	Breakfast	AM SNACK	Lunch	PM SNACK	Dinner
Day 1	Two scrambled eggs, spinach, and egg white	A fruit and sunflower seeds	Olive Oil over salad (salmon, bell peppers, kale, and cucumbers)	Asparagus spears	Grilled breast chicken over tomato sauce and zucchini noodles
Day 2	Cottage cheese, cinnamon, and slivered almonds	Hummus and sliced vegetables	Chicken (stir-fry) with brown rice and pepper	Peanut butter and sliced apple	Turkey tacos, lettuce and avocado slice
Day 3	Spinach, onions, and tomatoes in an egg frittata	Protein shake with fresh fruits	Salad with grilled chicken, tomato, tzatziki sauce, and garbanzo beans	Sliced veggies and hummus	Fish with olive oil, cauliflower, and roasted broccoli
Day 4	Delicious smoothie with berries, almond milk, and Greek yogurt	Hummus and chopped veggies	Veggie, avocado, and turkey sandwich on whole-wheat bread	Cubed cantaloupe and pistachios	Stir-fry steak on cauliflower rice
Day 5	Omelet with spinach, peppers, and avocado slices	Healthy protein bar	Quinoa with chopped chicken breast, vegetables, and vinaigrette	Peanut butter and carrots	Sautéed mushrooms, steamed broccoli, and salmon
Day 6	Hard-boiled two eggs and blueberries	Sliced almonds and Greek yogurt	Lentil salad, sun-dried tomatoes, raw vegetables, and kalamata olives	Healthy protein shake	Bean and vegetable soup with a grilled chicken

Day 7	Delicious Greek yogurt with walnuts, cinnamon, and apples	Sliced avocado and hard-boiled eggs	Shredded chicken stuffed in sweet potato with low-sugar sauce	Veggies and hummus	Veggie kabobs and shrimp with delicious cauliflower rice
Day 8	Pancakes	Roasted Almonds 7 to 8	Stuffed Bell Pepper	Handful Olives	Vegetable Chili
Day 9	Almond Milk, pancake	7 to 8 Toasted Cashews	Chicken Salad	Vegetable Rolls	Roasted Chicken
Day 10	Yogurt parfait and Smoothie of your choice	Almond Bars	Cauliflower Rice	Toasted Peanuts 7 to 8	Chicken pasta with salad
Day 11	Breakfast Muffins	1 Brownie	Chicken Fajita	Handful Strawberries	Beef soup
Day 12	Your Favorite Smoothie	Toasted Almonds 10	Apple Cake	Toasted Sunflower Seeds 7 to 8	Salmon cakes
Day 13	Savory brownies	Pumpkin Pie	Chicken Salad and Salsa	½ Avocado	Spinach soup
Day 14	Berry Smoothie	Toasted Almonds	Pumpkin soup	Apple sorbet	Shrimp Harissa
Day 15	Summer Squash and black beans	Bread with jalapeno spread	Tuna salad with cranberry	Handful Toasted Cashews	Balsamic Bruschetta and grilled chicken
Day 16	Pancakes	Toasted Sunflower Seeds	Beef Stew	Chickpea Salad	Chicken Fajita

Day 17	Tofu and smoothie	Mixed dried fruits	Roasted chicken and rice	Chicken Skewer	Lentil Sandwich and muffin
Day 18	Spinach omelet and smoothie	Toasted sesame seeds	Chinese soup	Pumpkin Seeds	Steak and vegetable chili
Day 19	Vegetable Frittata	Roasted Vegetables	Chicken Salad	Handful Nuts	Butter squash noodles and soup
Day 20	Porridge and pancake	Handful Cranberries	Tacos	Peanut bars	Fish fillet
Day 21	Omelet and avocado	Handful Toasted macadamia nuts	Vegetable Salad	Rice bars	Spinach Manicotti and salad
Day 22	Smoothie and herbal tea	Fruity chicken salad	Vegetable chili	½ apple and Avocado	Roasted Turkey and salad
Day 23	Vegetable Casserole	Handful Blueberries	Chicken and vegetable salad	Cheese bars	Chicken Stir-Fry
Day 24	Green Smoothie	Cornflakes cookies	Shrimp soup	Handful Toasted almonds	Salmon cake
Day 25	Muffins	Tofu bites	Chicken salad and nuts	Black beans salad	Salmon with soya beans
Day 26	Delicious smoothie	Guacamole	Salad and cauliflower rice	Coconut milk	Chicken soup
Day 27	Avocado, bread and eggs	Toasted almonds	Delicious chicken Salad	Gherkins Salad	Broil fish

Day 28	Pancakes and smoothie	Almond bars	Vegetable and fruit salad	Tahini and Carrot	Soup and noodles
Day 29	Omelet and bread	½ Avocado	Salad, Sandwich and stuffed dates	Smoothie	Chicken fillet and salad
Day 30	Cranberry Smoothie and toasted nuts	Sugar-free pie	Chicken Verde	Toasted Cashews	Roasted lamb

With the help of this sample diet plan, you can design a customized plan. Losing weight is not an easy task. Endomorph diet will help you to win this uphill battle and maintain a healthy weight. Understand your body type and unique challenges for endomorphs. It will help you to drop extra pounds and hit a fitness goal.

Breakfast Recipes

Recipe 01: Chicken Salad Wrap

Chicken salad wraps are healthy and delicious. It can be a yummy addition to your endomorph diet.

Preparation Time: 10 minutes

Total Time: 10 minutes

Servings: 6

Ingredients:

- 10 ounces of chicken chunks
- ¼ cup diced onion
- 4 tablespoons salsa
- ¼ cup mayonnaise
- Pepper and salt to taste
- 12 lettuce leaves
- 6 flour tortillas

Directions:

1. Take a bowl to combine the onion, chicken, salsa, mayonnaise, pepper, and salt in this bowl. Mix everything together.
2. Line every tortilla with only two lettuce leaves and divide chicken salad blend equally among every tortilla. Roll them up or carefully wrap. Salad wraps are ready to serve.

Nutritional Facts (Per Serving)

Calories: 463.7, Protein: 27.2 gram, Carbohydrates: 42.5 gram, Fat: 14.8 gram, Cholesterol: 61.4 mg, Sodium: 933.7mg and Cholesterol: 61.4mg

Recipe 02: Scrambled Eggs with Spinach

Start your day with scrambled eggs with spinach and tomatoes. It will be a delicious breakfast for everyone.

Preparation Time: 5 minutes

Cooking Time: 5 minutes

Servings: 2

Ingredients:

- 1 tablespoon rapeseed oil + 1 teaspoon oil
- 3 halved tomatoes
- 4 eggs
- 4 tablespoons yogurt
- 1/3 pack chopped basil
- 1 cup spinach (wash and dry well)

Directions:

1. Heat 1 teaspoon oil in a non-stick pan and add tomatoes in the oil. Cook them over medium heat (cut-side down). While the tomatoes are cooking, whisk eggs with yogurt in a bowl and mix in two tablespoons of water. Mix in sufficient basil and black pepper.
2. Transfer tomatoes to a serving plate and add spinach in the pan. Cook for a few minutes, let the spinach wilt and stir 2 to 3 times.
3. Pour remaining oil in the pan and heat it over medium flame. Pour in your egg mixture and stir consistently to scramble eggs. Spoon the spinach on your serving plate along with tomatoes and top with scrambled eggs.

Nutritional Value:

Calories: 297, Fat: 19 gram, Carbs: 10 grams, Protein: 20 grams, Salt: 0.6 grams, Fiber: 2 grams, Sugar: 10 grams

Recipe 03: Yummy Spinach Omelet

Get the essential vitamins and minerals of spinach. It will be the healthy start for a day.

Servings: 1

Preparation Time: 5 minutes

Total Time: 15 minutes

Ingredients:

- Eggs: 2
- Ground nutmeg: 1/8 teaspoon
- Chopped onion: ¼ teaspoon
- Torn Spinach leaves (baby spinach): 1 cup
- Pepper and salt: as per taste
- Parmesan cheese (grated): 1 ½ tablespoons

Instruction:

1. Whisk eggs in a bowl and mix in parmesan cheese and baby spinach. Season this blend with pepper, salt, nutmeg, and onion.

2. Grease one small skillet with olive oil or cooking spray over medium flame. Cook egg mixture for almost 3 minutes, until moderately set.

3. Flip egg with one spatula and continue cooking 2 – 3 minutes. Decrease heat to almost low and continue cooking again for 2 – 3 minutes. Serve hot.

Nutrition Value:

Calories: 186 kcal, Carbs: 2.8 g, Fat: 12.3 g, Protein: 16.4 g, Cholesterol: 379 mg, Sodium: 279 mg.

Recipe 04: Savory Brownies

Give a new twist to your brownies with this amazing recipe. It has several healthy and delicious ingredients.

Servings: 24

Preparation Time: 15 minutes

Total Time: 55 minutes

Ingredients:

- Chopped and rinsed spinach: 10 ounces
- Milk: 1 cup
- Melted butter: ½ cup
- All-purpose flour: 1 cup
- Chopped onion: 1
- Salt: 1 teaspoon
- Mozzarella cheese (shredded): 8 ounces
- Baking powder: 1 teaspoon
- Eggs: 2

Instruction:

1. Preheat your oven to almost 375 °F. Grease a baking dish (9x13-inch).

2. Put spinach in one medium saucepan with sufficient water to cover spinach. Let it boil and decrease heat to simmer. Cook for almost 3 minutes to limp spinach. Turn off heat. Drain spinach and keep it aside.

3. Take one large bowl and mix baking powder, salt and flour. Mix in butter, milk and eggs. Stir in mozzarella cheese, onion and spinach.

4. Transfer this mixture to your greased baking dish. Bake in your preheated oven for almost 30 – 35 minutes. Check with a toothpick, if it comes out clean, the brownies are ready.

Nutrition Value:

Calories: 92 kcal, Carbs: 5.6 g, Fat: 6 g, Protein: 4.1 g, Cholesterol: 32 mg, Sodium: 216 mg.

Recipe 05: Vegan Muffin

Banana, maple syrup and pecans make a delicious and healthy breakfast. You can enjoy it at the start of your day.

Servings: 12

Total Time: 45 minutes

Ingredients:

- Ripe bananas: 3
- Maple syrup: 1/2 cup
- Canola oil: 3 tablespoons
- Spelt flour: 1 1/2 cups
- Baking soda: 1 1/2 teaspoons
- Salt: 1/4 teaspoon
- Pecans: 3/4 cup

Instructions:

1. Preheat your oven to almost 350°F. Grease your muffin tins.

2. Take one bowl and mash bananas and mix in vanilla, canola oil and maple syrup.

3. Take another bowl and sift all dry ingredients together. Blend them with banana mixture and mix them well. Add pecans in the last and toss this mixture.

4. Pour into muffin tins and bake for almost 42 minutes. Check with a toothpick and serve.

Nutrition Value:

Calories: 451 kcal, Carbs: 59.2 g, Fat: 23.2 g, Protein: 4.1 g, Cholesterol: 0 mg, Sodium: 386 mg.

Recipe 06: Cauliflower Rice

Cauliflower has numerous health benefits. For weight loss, it will be an impressive addition to your diet.

Servings: 6

Total Time: 45 minutes

Ingredients:

- Cubed carrot: 1 large
- Frozen peas: 2 cups
- Minced garlic: 2 cloves
- Water: ½ cup
- Shredded cauliflower: 20 ounces
- Sesame oil (divided): ¼ cup
- Soy sauce: 6 tablespoons
- Whisked eggs: 2
- Sliced green onions: 6

Instruction:

1. Stir water and peas together in one saucepan and let it boil. Decrease heat to medium and cook for almost 5 minutes to tender peas. Drain and dispose of water.

2. Heat two tablespoons sesame oil in one wok over medium heat. Sauté garlic, carrot and onions in hot oil for almost 5 minutes to make them soft. Now add cauliflower, cook and mix until the cauliflower becomes tender. It will take almost 4 – 5 minutes.

3. Stir soy sauce and peas in cauliflower mixture and stir-fry this mixture for almost 3 – 5 minutes.

4. Move this mixture to side of wok and pour whisked eggs on empty side. Quickly scramble eggs for almost 3 – 5 minutes until heated through. Mix cooked eggs in cauliflower mixture and break up large chunks. Serve hot.

Nutrition Value:

Calories: 366 kcal, Carbs: 15.8 g, Fat: 19.2 g, Protein: 33.3 g, Cholesterol: 132 mg, Sodium: 1065 mg.

Recipe 07: Peach Smoothie

Servings: 1 to 2

Preparation Time: 5 minutes

Ingredients:

- Rinsed kale: 1 to 2 handfuls
- Peach: 1 pitted
- Banana: 1
- Strawberries: 1 handful
- Flax seeds: 1/8 cup
- Goji berries: 1/8 cup
- Water

Instructions:

1. Add all fruits and vegetables in a blender and add water to Max Line and extract all nutrients. You can enjoy a glass of extract nutrients with some ice.

Nutrition Value:

Calories: 105 kcal, Carbs: 38.5 g, Fat: 0.5 g, Protein: 6.3 g, Sodium: 34 mg.

Recipe 08: Green Smoothie

Servings: 1 to 2

Preparation Time: 5 minutes

Ingredients:

- Swiss chard (rinsed): 1 to 2 handfuls
- Apricot: 1
- Cored pineapple: 1 cup
- Apple: 1
- Blueberries: 1 cup
- Goji berries (soaked): ¼ cup
- Water

Instructions:

Add all fruits and vegetables in blender and add water to Max Line and extract all nutrients. You can enjoy a glass of extract nutrients with some ice.

Nutrition Value:

Calories: 204 kcal, Carbs: 48.5 g, Fat: 0.5 g, Protein: 4.3 g, Cholesterol: 2 mg, Sodium: 34 mg.

Recipe 09: Pineapple Smoothie

Servings: 1 to 2

Preparation Time: 5 minutes

Ingredients:

- Collard greens (rinsed): 1 to 2 handfuls
- Banana: 1
- Pineapple: 1 cup
- Red grapes: 1 cup
- Hemp seeds: ¼ cup
- Water

Instructions:

Add all fruits and vegetables in blender and add water to Max Line and extract all nutrients. You can enjoy a glass of extract nutrients with some ice.

Nutrition Value

Calories: 235 kcal, Carbs: 38.5 g, Fat: 1.5 g, Protein: 20.3 g, Cholesterol: 0 mg, Sodium: 143 mg.

Recipe 10: Beetroot Smoothie

Servings: 1 to 2

Preparation Time: 5 minutes

Ingredients:

- Raw beet: ¼
- Red grapes without seeds: 10
- Broccoli florets: 2 small
- Raspberries: 10
- Goji berries: 1 tablespoon
- Small avocado (peeled and pitted): ½
- Olive oil: 1 teaspoon

Instructions:

Add all fruits, olive oil and vegetables in blender and add water to Max Line and extract all nutrients. You can enjoy a glass of extract nutrients with some ice.

Nutrition Value:

Calories: 256 kcal, Carbs: 41.5 g, Fat: 0.7 g, Protein: 3.3 g, Cholesterol: 1 mg, Sodium: 32 mg.

Recipe 11: Kale Smoothie

Servings: 1 to 2

Preparation Time: 5 minutes

Ingredients:

- Kale: 2 handfuls
- Blueberries: 1 cup
- Banana: ½
- Cooked oatmeal: ⅓ cup
- Almonds: 10
- Raw cacao: 2 tablespoons

Instructions:

Add all fruits, nuts and vegetables in blender and add water to Max Line and extract all nutrients. You can enjoy a glass of extract nutrients with some ice.

Nutrition Value:

Calories: 261 kcal, Carbs: 38.5 g, Fat: 1.5 g, Protein: 9.3 g, Cholesterol: 0 mg, Sodium: 39 mg.

Recipe 12: Almond Chocolate Milk

Cooking Time: 5 minutes

Servings: 2 servings

Ingredients:

- Almond milk (unsweetened): 16 ounces
- Low-carb sweetener: to taste
- Heavy cream: 4 ounces
- Whey chocolate powder: 1 scoop
- Crushed ice: ½ cup

Instructions:

Put all above mentioned ingredients in your blender and blend them well to make a smooth paste. Serve chilled.

Nutrition: Calories: 292, Fat: 25 grams, Carbs: 5 and Protein: 15 grams

Recipe 13: Protein Berry Smoothie

Cooking Time: 10 minutes

Servings: 2 to 4

Ingredients:

- 2/3 cups berries
- Whey protein, 1 scoop
- ¼ cup water
- 1 cup chocolate milk
- 2 egg yolks, raw only

Instructions:

It is very simple, just take a full-size cup, blend all the ingredients and add crushed ice. You are done to enjoy your favorite chocolate bombs.

Nutrition Value:

279 total calories, 5.4 g fat, 9.7 g protein, 50.6 g carbohydrate, 122 mg sodium, 20 mg cholesterol

Recipe 14: Strawberry Smoothie

Cooking Time: 5 to 10 minutes

Servings: 2

Ingredients:

- Almond milk, 1 cup
- 2 tablespoons crushed almonds
- 1/3 cup strawberries
- One pinches salt

Instructions:

Take a food processor and make a blend of all these ingredients to make a delicious smoothie. Serve chilled by keeping in the refrigerator.

Nutritional Information:

840 total calories, 70 g fat, 27 g protein, 27 g carbohydrate and 2 g fiber.

Recipe 15: Blueberry Smoothie

Cooking Time: 10 minutes

Servings: 2

Ingredients:

- Almond milk, 1 cup
- 2 tablespoons crushed almonds
- 1/3 cup blueberries or any other berries of your choice
- One pinch salt

Instructions:

Take a food processor and make a blend of all these ingredients to make a delicious smoothie. Serve chilled by keeping in the refrigerator.

Nutritional Value:

835 total calories, 80 g fat, 30 g protein, 27 g carbohydrate and 2 g fiber.

Recipe 16: Yummy Quiche

Total Time: 30 minutes

Servings: 4

Ingredients:

- 3 organic eggs
- 4 organic egg whites
- 5 quartered cherry tomatoes
- 2/3 cup chopped asparagus, chop into 1-inch pieces
- 1/3 cup chopped bell pepper, green
- ½ cup mozzarella cheese, shredded
- Pepper and salt to taste

Directions:

1. Whisk whole eggs and egg white in a bowl until smooth, keep aside.
2. Chop bell peppers, tomatoes, asparagus, and mix into whisked egg bowl.
3. Stir in only half of the parmesan cheese.
4. Use some olive oil to grease one pie dish and transfer egg mixture in this dish.
5. Top egg mixture with remaining cheese and bake at 350°F for almost 35 to 40 minutes.

Recipe 17: Egg Scrambled and Vegetables

Total Time: 15 minutes

Servings: 6

Ingredients:

- 3 cups baby spinach, organic
- 6 organic large eggs
- ½ diced red onion, organic
- 1 organic diced tomato
- 1 clove minced and crushed garlic
- 1 teaspoon pink salt
- 1 teaspoon black pepper, cracked
- ½ cup cheddar cheese, organic
- 1 ½ tablespoon olive oil, extra virgin

Directions:

1. Whisk eggs together in a bowl. Mix in salt and black pepper and keep aside.
2. Heat olive oil in a large pan. Ad in garlic, onion, spinach, tomato, and sauté for almost 5 to 7 minutes to cook veggies.
3. Pour whisked eggs over sautéed veggies and cook for extra 3 to 4 minutes. Stir occasionally and cook to set eggs.
4. Turn off heat and sprinkle eggs with some cheese. Serve hot.

Recipe 18: Yogurt Parfait

Total Time: 10 minutes

Servings: 1

Ingredients:

- 1 cup Greek Yogurt, non-fat
- 1 packet Splenda
- ½ teaspoon organic vanilla extract
- 8 pretzels of any brand
- 10 chopped strawberries

Directions:

1. Put all pretzels in a plastic zip bag and use a mallet to smash them.
2. Layer the yogurt, pretzels and strawberries. You can make 2 to 3 layers. Serve.

Recipe 19: Yogurt Pancakes

Total Time: 20 minutes

Servings: 14

Ingredients:

- 1 cup all-purpose flour
- 2 cups plain Greek yogurt, nonfat
- 2 teaspoons baking soda
- 4 whisked eggs
- 1 teaspoon salt
- ½ cup low-fat 1% milk
- 1 teaspoon vanilla

Directions:

1. Take a medium mixing bowl and pour yogurt into this bowl. Combine remaining dry ingredients and mix into yogurt. Stir well until dry ingredients are completely incorporated in the yogurt.
2. Combine vanilla, milk, and eggs. Add this blend to yogurt blend and mix well to combine.
3. Grease a griddle pan or skillet and pour ½-cup batter to make a pancake of 5-inch diameter. Cook for 2 minutes to make its one side golden brown. Now flip this pancake when bubbles appear on the uncooked side. Cook this side for 1 to 2 minutes until golden brown.
4. Replicate this procedure with remaining batter to make almost 14 pancakes. Serve hot with your favorite syrup.

Recipe 20: Cheese Casserole

Total Time: 30 minutes

Servings: 4

Ingredients:

- ¼ cup shredded cheddar cheese, fat free
- 6 organic eggs
- 4 chopped turkey sausages
- ¼ cup chopped cherry tomatoes
- ½ chopped red onion
- ½ red or green bell pepper
- ¼ cup chopped mushrooms
- Garlic salt, to taste
- Pepper, to taste
- Red pepper flakes, to taste
- Oregano, to taste

Directions:

1. Crack eggs in one bowl and whisk well.
2. Add cheese, sausages, cherry tomatoes, red onion, bell pepper, mushrooms, garlic salt, pepper, red pepper flakes and oregano in whisked eggs.
3. Mix well and transfer this blend to a greased casserole dish.
4. Bake this blend for almost 35 minutes at 350°F or until cooked through. Serve hot.

Recipe 21: Oatmeal Muffins

Total Time: 40 minutes

Servings: 12

Ingredients:

- 1 egg
- 2 mashed bananas, medium
- 1 teaspoon vanilla
- 1/3 cup skim milk
- 1 teaspoon baking powder
- 2 ¼ cup large flake Quaker oats
- ½ teaspoon cinnamon
- Raspberry, apricot or mixed fruit jam without sugar

Directions:

1. Preheat your oven to 350°F. Spray 12 muffin tins with non-stick cooking spray.
2. Whisk egg and milk together in a bowl. Mix in vanilla and mashed banana.
3. Mix in cinnamon, baking powder, and oats.
4. Divide batter between 12 greased muffin cups. Make an indent in the center of each muffin to add jam. Drop ½ to 1 tablespoon of jam in each muffin.
5. Bake for almost 22 minutes in your preheated oven.
6. You can store these muffins in the fridge for a few days.

Recipe 22: Cinnamon and Apple Toast

Total Time: 55 minutes

Servings: 4

Ingredients:

- 2 diced and peeled apples
- 8 medium-sized slices of brown bread
- 4 eggs
- 2 teaspoons cinnamon
- 1 1/3 cup egg whites
- 1 cup milk, 1%

Directions:

1. Preheat your oven to exactly 350°F. Spray one casserole dish (9x13) with non-stick cooking spray.
2. Mix 1-teaspoon cinnamon and diced apples in a bowl (microwave safe). Cover this bowl tightly with saran wrap and put in the microwave for almost 3 minutes. Stir well.
3. Spread four slices of bread in a dish and equally top all slices with apples. Put the remaining four slices over the apples to make healthy sandwiches.
4. Take a bowl to whisk egg whites and egg together. Mix in milk and 1-teaspoon cinnamon. Pour this mixture over bread sandwiches to cover them well. The mixture can spread in the dish, but don't worry because it will be the part of serving.
5. Bake sandwiches in the oven for almost 45 minutes to cook eggs.
6. Serve with sugar-free syrup. Keep it in mind that two tablespoons of syrup will be equal to 1 smart freestyle points.

Lunch Recipes

Recipe 23: Chicken Parmesan

Total Time: 30 minutes

Servings: 4

Ingredients:

- 1 pound skinless and boneless chicken cutlets
- ¼ cup breadcrumbs, panko
- 1 whisked egg
- ¼ cup parmesan cheese, grated
- 1 teaspoon Italian seasoning
- 1 teaspoon garlic powder
- Pepper and salt, as per taste
- 2 teaspoons olive oil
- 3 cups fresh green beans
- ½ cup spicy marinara sauce
- ¼ cup chopped fresh basil
- ½ cup mozzarella cheese, shredded

Directions:

1. Preheat your oven to 425°F. Spray a non-stick baking sheet with a cooking spray.
2. Combine pepper, salt, Italian seasoning, garlic powder, parmesan cheese, and panko breadcrumbs in a bowl.
3. Press a side of chicken in the whisked egg and the parmesan and panko mixture. Put this chicken slice over a baking sheet with breading up. Replicate this process with remaining slices of chicken. If you want to increase the crispy texture of chicken, spray it with some olive oil.
4. Toss green beans with olive oil and sprinkle some pepper and salt as per taste. Spread out these beans around chicken over a baking sheet.
5. Cook for almost 15 minutes in your preheated oven to tender chicken. Remove pan from oven and top each chicken piece with mozzarella cheese and marinara sauce. Return this baking dish in the oven to cook for 1 to 2 minutes.
6. Top with basil or mint and serve hot.

Recipe 24: Mushroom Chicken

Total Time: 25 minutes

Servings: 4

Ingredients:

- 1.33 pounds skinless and boneless chicken breast
- 8 oz. sliced mushrooms
- 2 teaspoons olive oil
- 2 minced garlic cloves
- ½ cup chicken broth, low-sodium
- 1 ½ tablespoons balsamic vinegar
- Pepper and salt, to taste
- 1 tablespoon chopped parsley
- ½ teaspoon thyme

Directions:

1. Use pepper and salt to season chicken. Heat olive oil in a pan over medium heat. Add chicken in hot oil and carefully sear both sides of chicken for 2 to 3 minutes, until light brown. Remove chicken and keep aside.
2. Now add mushrooms and garlic to skillet and cook for 3 to 4 minutes to tender mushrooms.
3. Add thyme, balsamic vinegar, and chicken broth to your skillet. Mix and scrape browned chicken bits off the base of the skillet. Add chicken and simmer it for almost 10 to 15 minutes over low heat, until thoroughly cooked.

Recipe 25: Chicken Fajitas

Total Time: 40 minutes

Servings: 4

Ingredients:

- 1.33 lbs skinless and boneless chicken breast, chop into strips
- 1 sliced onion
- 14 ounces diced tomatoes and green chilies
- 1 sliced red pepper
- 1 sliced green pepper
- 2 teaspoons vegetable oil
- 1 cup sliced mushrooms
- 1 ½ teaspoon cumin
- 1 ½ teaspoon chili powder
- 1 teaspoon paprika
- ½ teaspoon onion powder
- ½ teaspoon garlic powder
- ½ teaspoon dried oregano
- ¼ teaspoon salt

Directions:

1. Preheat your oven to precisely 400°F.
2. Add each ingredient in a baking dish (glass dish) and toss everything with your hands. For your convenience, you can add chicken, veggies, and tomatoes. Sprinkle oil and spices on top and toss.
3. Bake for almost 25 to 30 minutes until cook through. Serve hot.

Recipe 26: Mouthwatering Fish Burgers

Total Time: 20 minutes

Servings: 4

Ingredients:

- ¼ cup Panko seasoned breadcrumbs
- 1 pound tilapia
- 1 egg white
- 1 egg
- 2 tablespoons Dijon Mustard
- 1 minced garlic clove
- 1 teaspoon salt
- 1 teaspoon onion powder
- ½ teaspoon black pepper
- 1 teaspoon paprika
- 1 teaspoon vegetable oil
- ½ teaspoon basil
- 4 hamburger buns, reduced calorie
- 1 sliced tomato
- I sliced cucumber
- ½ avocado

Directions:

1. Put fish in your food processor and pulse it to chop.
2. Combine chopped fish with egg white, egg, breadcrumbs, onion powder, basil, paprika, pepper, salt, garlic, and mustard.
3. Put this blend in a fridge for almost 10 minutes before making patties. After 10 minutes, form patties with this blend.
4. Brush all burgers with olive oil.
5. Grease a skillet and cook patties in this skillet over medium flame for almost 4 minutes each side.
6. Serve patties on toasted burger buns with tomato slices and avocado.

Recipe 27: Tasty Parmesan Shrimps with Garlic

Total Time: 15 minutes

Servings: 4

Ingredients:

- 2 tablespoons olive oil or melted butter
- 1.33 lbs deveined, peeled and raw shrimp
- 3 minced garlic cloves
- ¼ cup grated parmesan
- 1 teaspoon Italian seasoning
- 1 lime or lemon juice
- Pepper and salt, to taste

Directions:

1. Preheat your oven to precisely 300°F.
2. Toss all shrimps with parmesan cheese, Italian seasoning, garlic, and olive oil. Put tossed shrimps in one layer on your baking sheet.
3. Cook in your preheated oven for almost 6 to 8 minutes to cook through. Serve with lemon juice.

Recipe 28: Tuna Salad and Cranberry

Total Time: 10 minutes

Servings: 5

Ingredients:

- 3 tablespoons low-fat mayonnaise
- 16 ounces white tuna, water packed, drained
- 3 tablespoons sour cream, light
- ½ cup chopped celery
- ¼ cup minced red onion
- ¼ cup cranberries, dried
- 1 tablespoons lemon juice
- 1 diced apple
- Pepper and salt, to taste

Directions:

1. Take a bowl and combine mayonnaise, white tuna, sour cream, celery, red onion, cranberries, lemon juice, apple, salt, and pepper in this bowl.
2. Mix well and put in the fridge to serve chilled. You can eat right away.

Recipe 29: Summer Squash with Black Beans

Total Time: 50 minutes

Servings: 4

Ingredients:

- 2 cups black beans, drained and rinsed
- 4 zucchini or summer squash
- 1 minced garlic clove
- 1 cup minced onion
- ½ cup diced bell pepper, red
- ½ teaspoon cumin
- ½ cup shredded reduced fat cheddar cheese
- 1 cup red enchilada sauce

Directions:

1. Preheat your oven to precisely 400°F.
2. Take summer squash and scoop out its middle. Chop the scooped out squash to make it a part of your filling.
3. Put a skillet over medium heat and add onion, scooped out pieces of squash, bell pepper, garlic and black beans in the skillet. Cook for almost 5 to 7 minutes to tender.
4. Stir in pepper, salt, and cumin. Add enchilada sauce to the mixture.
5. Fill every summer squash with this blend and put in the baking dish. Sprinkle each squash with cheese.
6. Cover the baking dish with a foil and put in a preheated oven to bake for almost 25 minutes. After this time, remove foil and bake again for 10 minutes.

Recipe 30: Chicken Pasta

Total Time: 40 minutes

Servings: 8

Ingredients:

- 12 ounces penne pasta
- 2 cups cubed or shredded chicken
- 8 ounces cream cheese, fat-free
- ½ cup hot sauce
- ½ cup sour cream, fat-free
- 1 ounce ranch seasoning blend
- 1 cup cheddar cheese, fat-free and divided

Directions:

1. Preheat your oven to precisely 375°F.
2. Cook pasta as per the instructions on the package, drain and keep aside.
3. Grease a casserole dish with a nonstick spray.
4. Take a bowl and mix cheese (1/2 cup), sour cream, ranch mix, hot sauce, cream cheese and chicken in this bowl. Stir in drained pasta.
5. Pour this blend in a casserole dish and equally spread this mixture.
6. Top it with remaining fat-free cheese and bake for almost 18 to 20 minutes to melt cheese and heat through. Serve hot.

Recipe 31: Spinach Manicotti

Total Time: 30 minutes

Servings: 8

Ingredients:

- 15 ounces ricotta cheese, skim
- 16 crespelles, homemade (see bonus recipes)
- 1 organic large egg
- 2 cups mozzarella cheese, shredded (reserve half cup)
- 10 ounces fresh peas
- ½ teaspoon pink salt
- ¼ cup parmesan regianno, grated
- 2 ½ cups marinara sauce (see bonus recipes)
- Black pepper, as per taste

Directions:

1. Make crespelles.
2. Preheat your oven to precisely 375°F.
3. Take a bowl and combine 1 ½ cups of mozzarella, ricotta, spinach, egg, parmesan cheese, pepper and salt (1/2 teaspoon) in this bowl.
4. Fill every crespelle with spinach filling (almost ¼ cup) and roll.
5. Take a baking dish (you can take two as per your need) and pour 1 cup sauce on its base. Put manicotti rolled (seem area down) on the baking dish. Top with remaining mozzarella cheese and 1 ½ cups sauce.
6. Cover this dish with a foil and bake for almost 25 minutes, until bubbling and hot. Let the cheese melt. Serve hot.

Recipe 32: Potato Soup

Total Time: 45 minutes

Servings: 10

Ingredients:

- 1 diced carrot
- 2 cups cubed potatoes
- 2 thinly sliced leeks
- 1-tablespoon extra-virgin olive oil
- 1 diced onion
- 4 cups chicken or vegetable broth
- 2 cups pure rice milk
- 2 cups fresh water
- ½ cup potato flakes
- 3 minced garlic cloves
- 2 tablespoons butter
- 2 tablespoons ground black pepper
- 2 tablespoons salt
- 1 teaspoon fine garlic powder
- 1 teaspoon fine onion powder
- 1 teaspoon paprika, smoked

Directions:

1. Take a stockpot (6-quart) and put on high heat. Add olive oil, garlic, carrots, leeks, and onions in the crockpot. Cook for almost 5 minutes, stir regularly to tender vegetables.
2. Mix in potatoes, milk, water, and broth. Let this mixture boil
3. Decrease heat to medium, add potatoes flakes, seasonings, and butter in the crockpot.
4. Continue cooking for almost 20 to 25 minutes, stir occasionally.
5. Taste to adjust seasoning as per your desire.
6. Serve potato soup with green onions, bacon, and dairy-free shredded cheese.

Recipe 33: Apricot BBQ Chicken

Total Time: 35 minutes

Servings: 6

Ingredients:

- ½ cup apricot jam, sugar-free
- 1-pound skinless and boneless chicken breasts
- ½ cup BBQ Sauce, sugar-free
- 1 teaspoon ginger powder
- 1 teaspoon dry onion powder
- 1 teaspoon dry garlic powder
- 2 tablespoons soy sauce, low sodium

Directions:

1. Take a bowl and mix the seasonings, soy sauce, BBQ sauce and jam together.
2. Use a foil to line one baking sheet and put chicken breasts over foil in the equal layer.
3. Now pour BBQ sauce over meat to cover each piece of chicken.
4. Bake at 350°F for almost 30 minutes.
5. Take out the chicken and serve with salad.

Recipe 34: Chicken Sautéed Rice

Total Time: 28 minutes

Servings: 6

Ingredients:

- 4 egg whites
- Cooking spray
- ½ cup raw chopped scallion, white and green parts
- 12 ounces raw skinless and boneless chicken breast, chop into cubes
- 2 cloves minced garlic cloves
- ½ cup diced uncooked carrots
- 2 cups regular long-grain brown rice, cooked
- 3 tablespoons soy sauce, low sodium
- ½ cup green peas

Directions:

1. Coat a nonstick pan with sufficient cooking spray. Put this pan over medium heat. Add whisked egg whites and cook well to scramble for almost 3 – 5 minutes. Stir frequently, remove from pan and keep aside.
2. Turn off heat, coat skillet again with sufficient cooking spray and put again over medium flame. Add garlic and scallions and sauté for two minutes. Add carrots and chicken, sauté to make chicken golden brown. Cook for almost 5 minutes.
3. Mix in scrambled egg whites, peas, soy sauce and brown rice (cooked). Stir twice for almost 1 minute. Serve hot.

Recipe 35: Tasty Chili

Total Time: 40 minutes

Servings: 10

Ingredients:

- 30 ounces kidney beans (rinsed and drained)
- 30 ounces pinto beans (rinsed and drained)
- 30 ounces black beans (rinsed and drained)
- 1 pound lean ground chicken
- 30 ounces Diced Tomatoes and Green Chilies
- ½ tablespoon oregano
- ½ tablespoon cumin
- 1 tablespoon chili powder
- 2 to 3 minced garlic cloves
- 1 diced onion
- 1 quartered lime
- 15 ounces tomato sauce

Directions:

1. Put ground meat in instant pot, use brown or sauté function to cook meat.
2. Pour remaining ingredients into instant pot other than lime. Quarter one lime and gently squeeze its juice in the pot. Throw the skin away.
3. Choose Meat/Stew or Beans/Chili button on the instant pot. Start your pot and carefully close it pressure valve. You have to cook for almost 20 to 35 minutes as per your instant pot.
4. After this time, carefully release the pressure of cooker, garnish with thyme and serve.

Recipe 36: Yummy Chicken Fajita

Total Time: 40 minutes

Servings: 4

Ingredients:

- 1 sliced onion
- 1 pound skinless and boneless lean chicken breasts, chop into strips
- 1 sliced bell pepper
- 1 cubed ripe tomato
- 2 teaspoons dry garlic powder
- 1 tablespoon ground cumin
- 1 teaspoon dry onion powder
- 1 teaspoon ground black pepper
- 1 teaspoon pink salt
- ½ teaspoon or more chili powder

Directions:

1. Preheat your oven to 375°F.
2. Spray a casserole dish with olive oil.
3. Mix seasoning together in a bowl.
4. Chop chicken into 1-inch bite-sized strips or pieces and coat them well with some seasoning blend.
5. Spread seasoned chicken pieces in a layer in the base of greased casserole dish.
6. Top chicken with vegetables. Bake at precisely 375°F for 35 to 40 minutes to brown vegetables.
7. Serve with tomato, lettuce, sour cream, guacamole, cheese, salsa, and tortillas.

Recipe 37: Baked Salmon

Total Time: 20 minutes

Servings: 4

Ingredients:

- 3 minced garlic cloves
- 2 pounds salmon
- ¼ cup chopped parsley
- Salt, to taste
- ½ cup shredded parmesan cheese

Directions:

1. Preheat your oven to 425°F.
2. Line your baking sheet with a parchment paper.
3. Season salmon filet with salt to taste.
4. Put salmon filet (skin-side down) on the parchment paper. Cover it with another parchment paper. Put fish in the oven to bake for almost 10 minutes.
5. Blend the minced garlic, parmesan cheese and chopped parsley in a bowl.
6. Take out salmon from oven and discard the top parchment paper.
7. Top salmon with herb mixture and put in the oven again. Cook for extra five minutes until done.
8. Take out from oven and wait for five minutes, serve hot.

Recipe 38: Chicken Nuggets

Total Time: 30 minutes

Servings: 4

Ingredients:

- ½ cup whole wheat or all-purpose flour
- 1 pound skinless and boneless chicken breasts
- 20 mini pretzels or pretzel sticks
- ¼ cup milk, skim
- ½ teaspoon black pepper
- 1 teaspoon garlic powder
- ¼ cup brown spicy mustard

Directions:

1. Preheat your oven to 400°F.
2. Add pretzels in a zippered plastic bag and seal. Crush them with the help of one rolling pin, food processor or heavy glass.
3. Use three shallow containers for the creation of dredging station.
4. Put flour with garlic and pepper in a container. Put mustard and milk in another container. Put crushed pretzels in the final container.
5. Chop chicken into small bite-sized pieces.
6. Dredge pieces of chicken in flour, mustard and finally in the pieces of pretzel.
7. Put on one baking sheet and bake for almost 20 to 23 minutes to make nuggets. Serve hot.

Recipe 39: Chicken Verde

Total Time: 6 hours

Servings: 6

Ingredients:

- 2 seeded jalapenos
- 1 pound chicken breasts without skin and bone
- ½ white quartered onion
- 6 quartered and peeled tomatillos
- 2 minced garlic cloves
- ½ cup low sodium and fat-free chicken broth
- ½ teaspoon pink salt
- 1 teaspoon cumin seeds
- ¼ teaspoon ground black pepper

Directions:

1. Puree jalapenos, quartered onion, tomatillos, garlic clove, pink salt, cumin seeds, ground black pepper and chicken broth in a blender to make it slightly chunky.
2. Put chicken in the base of the crockpot and add puree over chicken.
3. Cook this blend over low heat for almost 6 hours.
4. Shred chicken after six hours and serve with additional sauce over it.

Recipe 40: Chickpea Salad

Total Time: 10 minutes

Servings: 8

Ingredients:

- 30 ounces rinsed and drained chickpea
- 1 chopped tomato
- ½ teaspoon brown sugar
- ¼ cup chopped onion
- ¼ cup feta cheese, crumbled and reduced fat
- ½ tablespoon red vinegar
- ½ tablespoon fresh lemon juice
- 2 minced garlic cloves
- ¼ teaspoon pepper
- ¼ teaspoon salt
- 1 to 2 tablespoons cilantro
- 1 tablespoon Greek Yogurt

Directions:

1. Drain chickpeas and rinse thoroughly. Put them in a bowl.
2. Toss in tomato, brown sugar, onion, cheese, vinegar, lemon juice, garlic, pepper, salt, cilantro, and yogurt. Mix all ingredients well.
3. Now serve instantly and put the leftover in your fridge. You can secure it for a few days in your refrigerator.

Recipe 41: Grilled Shrimps

Total Time: 20 minutes

Servings: 5

Ingredients:

- 2 tablespoons vinegar, balsamic
- 24 deveined and clean medium shrimp
- 1 lemon, for juice
- 1 teaspoon coconut or olive oil
- 1 clove minced garlic
- ½ teaspoon black pepper
- ½ teaspoon salt
- 1 pinch flakes of red pepper

Sauce:

- 1 tablespoon Greek Yogurt
- 2 tablespoons tomato ketchup
- 1 tablespoon horseradish prepared sauce

Directions:

1. Take a bowl and mix together pepper flakes, pepper, salt, garlic, lemon juice, oil, and vinegar together.
2. Pour this blend over shrimp and cover shrimps to put in the fridge for almost 30 minutes.
3. Slide all shrimps (one by one) on skewers.
4. Carefully grill every side for 2 to 3 minutes. Shrimps take less time to cook so keep an eye on them when they turn pink and curl.

Sauce:

1. Take a bowl and mix ketchup, Greek yogurt, and horseradish sauce. You can increase or decrease horseradish sauce as per your taste.

Recipe 42: Cod Fillets

Servings: 4

Cooking Time: 2 hours for preparation

15 to 20 minutes for cooking

Ingredients:

- 2 raw scallions, crushed
- 1 Tablespoon ginger paste
- 2 teaspoons garlic paste
- 1 Tablespoon sherry cooking wine (non-alcoholic)
- 1 Tablespoon Soy sauce (reduced salt)
- 1.5 pounds raw Pacific cod

Directions:

1. Keep the fish in a baking dish. Take a small bowl and mix ginger, scallions, garlic, sherry and Soy sauce (reduced salt) to pour over the fish. Let it marinate for almost 2 hours.
2. Take a saucepan and fill it with water to keep on a high heat. Let it boil and keep fish in a steamer basket. Now discard marinade and keep the steamer basket in the saucepan. The basket should sit above water.
3. Steam fish after covering the saucepan and wait for its complete cooking. It should be easy to flake with a fork. It will take almost 10 minutes. Divide into pieces and enjoy.

Recipe 43: Grilled Chicken

Servings: 6

Cooking Time: 3 Hours for Marination and rest of the time in grilling and baking

Ingredients:

- 1.5 lbs. chicken breasts, 6 fillets (no skin and bone)
- 1 tablespoons sesame oil
- 1 cup cilantro
- 2 tablespoons Soy sauce (reduced salt), low sodium
- Juice from 1 lime
- 6 garlic cloves
- 1/2 cup chicken broth, fat-free
- 1 teaspoon salt
- 1/2 teaspoon black pepper powder

Directions:

1. Process all ingredients except chicken in the food processor to make them smooth. Now keep the chicken in a large bowl and pour blended mixture over the chicken.
2. It should cover all the chicken and now keep it in the refrigerator for almost 3 hours.
3. Prepare a grill and cook it until the temperature reaches 165F, use a meat thermometer. Keep the breasts on the grill for 5 minutes before enjoying it. Your one serving size will be one chicken breast.

Recipe 44: Chinese Soup

Cooking Time: One hour

Servings: 5

Ingredients:

- 14 oz. coconut milk, light
- 5 cups chicken broth, fat-free
- 1 tablespoon ginger, crushed
- 4 tablespoons fish sauce
- 1/4 cup lemongrass, chopped
- 2 tablespoons sauce (Siracha)
- Two limes, juice
- 2 tablespoons sugar
- 1/4 cup chopped scallions
- 1 cup peas, (sugar snap)
- 1/4 cup chopped cilantro
- 1/2 cup broccoli florets
- 2 zucchini, diced
- 1/3 cup carrots, sliced
- 1 cup mushrooms, chopped

Directions:

1. Take a large pot and add lemon grass, ginger and stock to let it boil. Keep it on a medium heat and cook for 30 minutes. Wait for lemongrass to release yummy flavors. Now add the lime juice, milk, both sauces, and sugar. Cook it for almost 10 minutes.
2. Meanwhile, blanch zucchini, broccoli and carrots in boiling water for almost 2 minutes. You have to make them a bit soft.
3. Now take 6 bowls and equally divide vegetables. Distribute soups equally into each bowl with the vegetables. Serve with cilantro as a topping.

Recipe 45: Baked Red Pepper

Cooking Time: One Hour

Servings: 3

Ingredients:

- 4 Red Bell Peppers
- 3 tablespoons bread crumbs, Italian seasoned
- 3 tablespoons grated cheese

Directions:

1. Preheat your oven to 350 degrees F or 175 C. Grease a nonstick cooking pan and set aside.
2. Slice bell peppers in half and removes its seeds and inner material. Now keep these slices in the prepared baking pan.
3. Prepare a mixture of cheese and breadcrumbs in a bowl. Sprinkle this mixture evenly on peppers. Bake it for 35 to 45 minutes to make the topping brown. Serve with your favorite healthy sauce.

Recipe 46: Balsamic Bruschetta

Cooking Time: 15 minutes

Servings: 8

Ingredients:

- Olive oil: 1 teaspoon
- Kosher salt: ¼ teaspoon
- Chopped fresh basil: 1/3 cup
- Diced tomatoes (Roma plum): 8
- Parmesan cheese (shredded): ¼ cup
- Ground black pepper: ¼ teaspoon
- Sliced and toasted bread: 1 loaf
- Minced garlic: 2 cloves
- Balsamic vinegar: 1 tablespoon

Directions:

1. Toss together garlic, parmesan cheese, basil and tomatoes in a bowl. Stir in balsamic vinegar, pepper, kosher salt, and olive oil.
2. Serve it on toasted bread slices.

Recipe 47: Guacamole

Cooking Time: 50 minutes

Servings: 16

Ingredients:

- Chopped jalapeno peppers: 2
- Avocados (pitted, peeled and diced): 2
- Fresh chopped cilantro: ½ tablespoon
- Salt: 2 teaspoons
- Lime juice: 2 tablespoons
- Diced tomato: 1
- Diced onion: 1

Directions:

1. Put avocados in a bowl along with salt and mash them. Mix well to equally distribute salt.
2. Stir in onion, tomato, lime juice, cilantro and jalapeno.
3. Cover this bowl and put in your fridge for 30 minutes. Serve chilled with taco or bread slices.

Recipe 48: Jalapeno Spread

Cooking Time: 13 minutes

Servings: 32

Ingredients:

- Jalapeno peppers (diced): 2 ounces
- Softened cream cheese: 16 ounces
- Parmesan grated cheese: 1 cup
- Mayonnaise: 1 cup
- Chopped green chilies: 4 ounces

Directions:

1. Stir mayonnaise and cream cheese together in a bowl to make this blend smooth. Mix in jalapeno peppers and green chilies.
2. Pour mixture in a microwave save dish and sprinkle with cheese.
3. Microwave for 3 minutes over high. Serve with tacos.

Recipe 49: Avocado Salad

Cooking Time: 8 hours 30 minutes

Servings: 32

Ingredients:

- Lemon juice: ¼ cup
- Corn kernels: 16 ounces
- Cider vinegar: 3 tablespoons
- Sliced ripe olives: 4.5 ounces
- Dried oregano: 1 teaspoon
- Chopped bell pepper (red): 1
- Salt: ½ teaspoon
- Chopped small onion: 1
- Ground black pepper: ½ teaspoon
- Minced garlic: 5 cloves
- Avocados (peeled, diced and pitted): 4
- Olive oil: 1/3 cup

Directions:

1. Take a bowl and mix onion, bell pepper, olives, and corn in this bowl.
2. Mix garlic, lemon juice, olive oil, salt, pepper, oregano, cider vinegar in a bowl. Pour in corn blend and toss well to coat.
3. Cover bowl and chill salsa in your fridge for 8 to 12 hours.
4. Stir avocadoes in this blend before serving.

Recipe 50: Roasted Vegetables

Cooking Time: 55 minutes

Servings: 12

Ingredients:

- Cubed butternut squash: 1
- Chopped thyme: 1 tablespoon
- Chopped rosemary: 2 tablespoons
- Diced and seeded red bell peppers: 2
- Cubed and peeled zucchini: 1
- Olive oil: ¼ cup
- Balsamic vinegar: 2 tablespoons
- Chopped Asparagus: 1 to 2 spears
- Ground black pepper and salt: to taste
- Quartered red onion: 1

Directions:

1. Preheat the oven to 475°F.
2. Combine zucchini, asparagus spears, bell peppers, and squash in a bowl. Separate onion quarters into pieces and add them to squash mixture.
3. Stir together pepper, salt, vinegar, olive oil, rosemary, and thyme in a bowl. Toss well with vegetables to coat them. Equally spread on a roasting pan.
4. Roast for almost 35 – 40 minutes in your preheated oven. Stir after every 10 minutes to make vegetables equally brown. Serve.

Recipe 51: Butter Squash Noodles

Butter squash is an amazing alternative of pasta. You can roast it quickly and make delicious noodles.

Preparation Time: 5 minutes

Total Time: 50 minutes

Servings: 4

Ingredients:

- Butternut squash noodles: 16 oz.
- Extra-virgin olive oil: 2 tablespoons
- Kosher salt: as per taste
- Ground black pepper: as per taste
- Red pepper crushed flakes: 1 Pinch
- Grated Parmesan: to serve

Directions:

1. Preheat your oven to almost 425° F. Put noodles on a baking sheet and toss them with salt, pepper, red pepper flakes and oil.
2. Roast for 10 minutes until golden and tender. Serve them warm with grated parmesan.

Nutritional Value:

Calories: 320kcal, Carbs: 30g, Protein: 10g, Saturated Fat: 4g, Sodium: 202mg, Iron: 2mg, Calcium: 266mg

Recipe 52: Fruity Chicken Salad

A tasty and healthy chicken salad with fruit and honey is best to eat the day after its preparation.

Preparation Time: 10 minutes

Cooking Time: 45 minutes

Servings: 8

Ingredients:

- Chicken breast, boneless, skinless halves (diced and cooked): 4
- Diced celery stalk: 1
- Chopped green onions: 4 medium
- Peeled and diced apple: 1
- Golden Raisins: 1/3 cup
- Halved green grapes (seedless): 1/3 cup
- Toasted chopped pecans: ½ cup
- Toasted black pepper (ground): 1/8 teaspoon
- Curry powder: ½ teaspoon
- Light mayonnaise: ¾ cup

Directions:

1. Take a large bowl and combine apple, raisins, onion, chicken, celery, pecans, grapes, curry powder, mayonnaise and pepper in this bowl.
2. Mix them well and serve.

Nutritional Value:

Calories: 229.2, Carbs: 12.3g, Protein: 15.1g, Fat: 14g (22% DV), Sodium: 188mg, Iron: 1 mg, Calcium: 25.9mg

Recipe 53: Nutty Chicken Salad

A rich, tasty and delicious cold salad with chicken and cream can be served on sandwiches and leaf.

Preparation Time: 20 minutes

Cooking Time: 20 minutes

Servings: 10

Ingredients:

- Chicken meat (cooked and diced): 2 ½ cups
- Chopped celery: 1 cup
- Seedless groups: 1 cup (sliced)
- Sliced almonds: ½ cup
- Chopped parsley: 2 tablespoons
- Salt: 1 tablespoon
- Mayonnaise: 1 cup
- Heavy whipping cream: ¼ cup

Directions:

1. Use a medium bowl to whip cream for soft peaks.
2. Combine almonds, grapes, parsley, celery, meat, mayonnaise and salt with whipped cream. Serve chilled.

Nutritional Value:

Calories: 274, Carbs: 5g, Protein: 11g, Fat: 23.6g, Sodium: 388mg, Iron: 0.5mg, Calcium: 30.5mg

Recipe 54: Black Beans Salad

This salad is loaded with copper, manganese, magnesium, zinc and calcium. It can build and maintain your bone strength and structure.

Cooking Time: 45 minutes

Servings: 6

Ingredients:

- Ground cumin: 2 teaspoons
- Olive oil: 2 tablespoons
- Cayenne pepper: ½ teaspoon
- Diced onion: 2 large
- Chopped garlic: 6 cloves
- Chopped green onions: ½ cup
- Black beans (drained and rinsed): 19 ounces
- Chopped cilantro: ¼ cup
- Tomato sauce: 16 ounces
- Chopped cilantro: ¾ cup
- Diced tomatoes: 2

Directions:

1. Heat coconut or olive oil in a pot over medium flame. Cook garlic and onion in oil for almost 5 – 7 minutes to tender.
2. Mix in cayenne pepper, cumin, diced tomatoes, tomato sauce and black beans. Decrease heat to medium and simmer for almost 5 minutes.
3. Mix ¾ cup of cilantro and simmer for another two minutes. Mix in green onion and turn off heat. Garnish with cilantro (1/4 cup) and serve.

Nutritional Value:

Calories: 464, Carbs: 52 g, Protein: 13 g, Fat: 24 g, Sodium: 591 mg, Fiber: 15 g

Recipe 55: Ricotta Pie with Swiss Chard

It can be a delicious choice for your lunch. You can consume this filling meal without any fear of gaining weight.

Preparation time: 10 minutes

Serves: 6

Ingredients:

- Olive oil: 1 tablespoon
- Chopped onion: ½ cup
- Garlic clove: 1
- Chopped swiss chard: 8 cups
- Whole milk ricotta cheese: 2 cups
- Eggs: 3
- Shredded mozzarella: 1 cup
- Shredded parmesan: ¼ cup
- Ground nutmeg: 1/8 teaspoon
- Salt: a pinch
- Pepper: a pinch
- Mild sausage: 1 lbs.

Directions:

1. Heat olive oil in a pan.
2. Fry chopped onion and minced garlic clove. Now add in the chopped swiss chard and fry until the leaves are wilted and the stems have become tender.
3. Mix in the ground nutmeg and season with salt and pepper. Set it aside.
4. Beat eggs in another bowl and add in whole milk ricotta cheese, parmesan cheese and the mozzarella cheese. Add in the fried Swiss chard mixture.
5. Roll out your sausage and press it in the pie tart and put in the prepared filling.
6. Preheat your oven at 350 degrees Fahrenheit and put your pie in oven for almost 25 to 30 minutes. You can add in more cheese if you wish to.

Nutritional Value:

Calories: 344, Fat: 27 grams, Protein: 23 grams, Carbs: 4 grams

Recipe 56: Yummy Pumpkin Bread

Pumpkin has several health benefits; therefore, it can be a suitable meal for breakfast and lunch.

Total Time: 1 hour

Servings: 24

Ingredients:

- Sugar: 3 cups
- Vegetable oil: 1 cup
- Eggs: 4
- Water: 2/3 cup
- Pumpkin puree: 15 ounces
- Ground ginger: 2 teaspoons
- Ground allspice: 1 teaspoon
- Ground cinnamon: 1 teaspoon
- Ground cloves: 1 teaspoon
- All-purpose flour: 3 1/2 cups
- Baking soda: 2 teaspoons
- Salt: 1 1/2 teaspoons
- Baking powder: 1/2 teaspoon

Directions:

1. Preheat your oven to 350°F. Lightly grease 2 loaf pans (9x5-inch).

2. Take a mixing bowl and combine eggs, oil and sugar in this bowl to make a smooth blend. Add some water and whisk to make a smooth blend. Mix in clove, cinnamon, allspice, ginger and pumpkin puree.

3. Take a medium bowl and combine baking powder, salt, soda and flour in this bowl. Add these dry ingredients to pumpkin blend and mix all ingredients well. Divide this batter between greased pans.

4. Bake these pans in preheated oven for almost 1 hour. Check with a toothpick, if it comes out dry, the bread is ready.

Nutritional Value:

Calories: 263.4, Carbs: 40.6 g, Protein: 11 g, Fat: 3.1 g, Sodium: 305.4 mg, Iron: 1 mg, Calcium: 28.5mg

Recipe 57: Lunch Casserole

You can enjoy a combination of bacon and eggs in the lunch. It will be a healthy meal to lose weight.

Total Time: 1 hour 15 minutes

Servings: 12

Ingredients:

- Sliced bacon: 1 pound
- Chopped sweet onion: 1
- Shredded hash brown frozen potatoes (thawed): 4 cups
- Lightly whisked eggs: 9
- Shredded Cheddar cheese: 2 cups
- Cottage cheese (small curd): 1 1/2 cups
- Swiss cheese (shredded): 1 1/4 cups

Directions:

1. Preheat your oven to almost 350°F. Grease one baking dish (9x13-inch).

2. Heat one skillet over medium heat and cook onion and bacon in the skillet for almost 10 minutes. Drain and transfer onion and bacon in one large bowl.

3. Mix in Swiss cheese, cottage cheese, cheddar cheese, eggs and potatoes. Pour this blend in a greased baking dish.

4. Put this baking dish in a preheated oven and bake for almost 45 – 50 minutes to melt cheese and set eggs. Keep baked eggs aside for almost 10 minutes before slicing and serving.

Nutritional Value:

Calories: 311.6, Carbs: 14.7 g, Protein: 15 g, Fat: 24 g, Sodium: 610.3 mg

Recipe 58: Tofu Bites

In your diet, tofu can be an excellent addition to increase protein. For weight loss, it has numerous amazing nutrients.

Total Time: 25 minutes

Servings: 4

Ingredients:

- Extra firm tofu: 16 ounce
- Soy sauce: 1/4 cup
- Maple syrup: 2 tablespoons
- Ketchup: 2 tablespoons
- Vinegar: 1 tablespoon
- Hot sauce: 1 dash
- Sesame seeds: 1 tablespoon
- Garlic powder: 1/4 teaspoon
- Ground black pepper: 1/4 teaspoon
- Liquid smoke flavoring: 1 teaspoon

Directions:

1. Preheat your oven to almost 375°F. Grease a non-stick baking sheet with the help of oil.
2. Make ½-inch slices of tofu and slowly press tofu slices to squeeze extra water of tofu. Cut tofu slices in ½-inch cubes.
3. Take a bowl and mix together hot sauce, vinegar, ketchup, maple syrup, and soy sauce in this bowl. Mix in liquid smoke, black pepper, garlic powder, and sesame seeds. Slowly mix tofu cubes in sauce. Cover this bowl and keep it aside for almost 5 minutes.
4. Put tofu on a baking sheet in one layer. Bake in your preheated oven for almost 15 minutes. Twist tofu and bake for almost 15 minutes to turn tofu golden brown.

Nutritional Value:

Calories: 176, Carbs: 6 g, Protein: 15 g, Fat: 10 g, Sodium: 614 mg, Iron: 2 mg, Calcium: 28.5mg

Recipe 59: Vegetable Chili

Vegetables are important for your diet. You can add your favorite vegetables in this recipe.

Total Time: 1 hour 10 minutes

Servings: 6

Ingredients:

- Chopped onions: 5
- Burger-style crumbles: 12 ounces
- Chili powder: 3 tablespoons
- Black beans (drained and rinsed): 30 ounces
- Ground cumin: 1 ½ tablespoons
- Red kidney beans (dark): 30 ounces
- Garlic powder: 1 tablespoon
- Red kidney beans (light): 15 ounces
- Bay leaves: 1 tablespoon
- Diced tomatoes: 29 ounces
- Tomato juice: 12 fluid oz.
- Pepper and salt: to taste

Directions:

1. Combine tomato juice, diced tomatoes, pepper, salt, bay leaves, kidney beans, black beans, garlic powder, cumin, chili powder, and onions in a pot.

2. Mix them well and let them simmer over medium heat for almost 1 hour. Cover the pot while cooking and serve hot chili.

Nutritional Value:

Calories: 236, Carbs: 37.6 g, Protein: 10.9 g, Fat: 3.1 g, Sodium: 305.4 mg, Iron: 1 mg, Calcium: 28.5 mg

Recipe 60: Bell Pepper

Total Time: 1 hour 10 minutes

Servings: 4

Ingredients:

- Chopper parsley: 2 tablespoons
- White rice (uncooked): ½ cup
- Tomato sauce: 2 cups
- Water: ¾ cup
- Mozzarella cheese (shredded): 4 ounces
- Bell peppers Green: 4
- Salt: to taste
- Chopped onion: 1
- Black pepper ground: to taste
- Olive oil: 4 tablespoons
- Vegetable protein (textured): 8 ounces

Directions:

1. Combine water and rice in a pan and let them boil. Decrease heat to almost low and simmer for almost 15 minutes.

2. Preheat your oven to almost 400°F.

3. Cut off the tops of peppers and remove seeds. Arrange peppers on a baking dish and chop usable part of the pepper's tops.

4. Heat oil in a skillet over medium flame. Sauté onion and chopped peppers in oil to make them soft. Mix in parsley and vegetable protein. Decrease heat to almost low and cook for 5 minutes. Stir in cooked rice and tomato sauce (1 1/5 cups).

5. Season with pepper and salt to taste. Spoon this blend in peppers and top every pepper with tomato sauce (remaining). Cover it and bake for almost 45 minutes. Remove cover, top every pepper with some mozzarella cheese and bake to melt. Serve hot.

Recipe 61: Roasted Bell Pepper and Tofu

Total Time: 1 hour 25 minutes

Servings: 2

Ingredients:

- Soy sauce: ¼ cup
- Extra firm tofu: 8 ounces (drained and cut into chunks)
- Zucchini (cut into chunks): 1
- Sesame oil: 2 tablespoons
- Diced onion: ¼ cup
- Red bell pepper (chop into chunks): 1
- Diced jalapeno pepper: 1
- Large mushrooms: 10
- Black pepper ground: to taste
- Chili garlic sriracha sauce: 2 tablespoons

Directions:

- Put mushrooms, red bell pepper, zucchini and tofu in one bowl. Mix pepper, jalapeno, onion, sesame oil, soy sauce, and sriracha sauce in one small bowl.

- Pour this blend over vegetables and tofu. Lightly toss tofu to coat and cover this blend. Put in the fridge for almost 1 hour.

- Preheat your outdoor grill for medium heat and grease the grate.

- Thread vegetables and tofu on to all skewers. Grill every skewer for 10 minutes or until done. You can use marinade as dipping sauce.

Dinner Recipes

Recipe 62: Roasted Turkey

Total Time: 4 hour 45 minutes

Servings: 16

Ingredients:

- Olive oil: ¾ cup
- Italian seasoning: 1 tablespoon
- Minced garlic: 3 tablespoons
- Ground black pepper: 1 teaspoon
- Salt: to taste
- Chopped rosemary: 2 tablespoons
- Whole turkey: 12 pounds
- Chopped basil: 1 tablespoon

Directions:

1. Preheat your oven to almost 325°F.

2. Mix olive oil, salt, black pepper, Italian seasoning, basil, rosemary, garlic and olive oil in a bowl. Keep this mixture aside.

3. Carefully wash turkey and remove extra fast deposits. Make skin loose from its breast. You can do this by working between breast and skin with your fingers. Work it loosely to end a drumstick, but don't tear the skin.

4. Spread sufficient amount of rosemary blend with the help of your hands beneath the leg, thigh and breast skin. Rub the remaining rosemary blend over the breast. You can seal skin with toothpicks over bare breast meat.

5. Put turkey on one rack in your roasting pan and add almost ¼-inch water to the base of a pan. Roast in your preheated oven for almost 3 – 4 hours or the internal temperature of the meat reaches 180°F.

Recipe 63: Roasted Pork

Total Time: 3 hours 20 minutes

Servings: 8

Ingredients:

- Sugar: ½ cup
- Rubbed sage: 1 teaspoon
- Cornstarch: 1 tablespoon
- Salt: ½ teaspoon
- Vinegar: ¼ cup
- Pepper: ¼ teaspoon
- Water: ¼ cup
- Crushed garlic: 1 clove
- Soy sauce: 2 tablespoons
- Boneless pork loin: 5 pounds

Directions:

1. Preheat your oven to almost 325°F.

2. Combine garlic, pepper, salt, and sage in one bowl. Rub this blend over pork. Put pork in a roasting pan (uncovered) in the center of your oven rack.

3. Bake in your preheated oven for almost 3 hours, until the temperature reaches to almost 145°F.

4. In the meantime, put water, soy sauce, vinegar, cornstarch and sugar in a saucepan. Heat and stir occasionally to bubble mixture and make it thick. Brush pork roast with glaze almost 3 – 4 times during last half hour. You can pour remaining glaze on the roast and serve hot.

Recipe 64: Beef Bulgogi

Total Time: 1 hour 15 minutes

Servings: 4

Ingredients:

- Thinly sliced flank steak: 1 pound
- Minced garlic: 2 tablespoons
- Sesame seeds: 2 tablespoons
- Soy sauce: 5 tablespoons
- Sesame oil: 2 tablespoons
- White sugar: 2 ½ tablespoons
- Black pepper ground: ½ teaspoon
- Chopped green onion: ¼ cup

Directions:

1. Put beef in one shallow dish. Combine black pepper, sesame oil, sesame seeds, garlic, green onion, sugar, and soy sauce in a bowl. Pour this blend over beef. Cover beef and put in the fridge for almost 1 hour or even whole night.
2. Preheat your outdoor grill for almost high heat and grease grate.
3. Quickly grill marinated beef over a hot grill for almost 1 – 2 minutes each side to cook through. Serve hot.

Recipe 65: BBQ Ribs

Total Time: 2 hours

Servings: 4

Ingredients:

- Salt: 2 tablespoons
- Pork ribs (country style): 2 ½ pounds
- Barbeque sauce: 1 cup
- Black pepper ground: 1 teaspoon
- Garlic powder: 1 tablespoon

Directions:

1. Put ribs in a pot with sufficient water to cover. Season with salt, black pepper, and garlic powder. Let this water boil and cook ribs to tender.

2. Preheat your oven to almost 325°F.

3. Remove cooked ribs from cooking pot and put them in a baking dish (9x13-inch). Pour whole barbeque sauce over cooked ribs. Cover this dish with an aluminum foil and bake for almost 1 – 1 ½ hours in your preheated oven. Serve hot.

Recipe 66: Roasted Lamb

Total Time: 40 minutes

Servings: 4

Ingredients:

- Frenched and trimmed rack of lamb: 7 bones
- Bread crumbs: ½ cup
- Salt: 1 teaspoon
- Minced garlic: 2 tablespoons
- Black pepper: 1 teaspoon
- Chopped rosemary: 2 tablespoons
- Olive oil: 2 tablespoons
- Salt: 1 teaspoon
- Dijon mustard: 1 tablespoon
- Black pepper: 1/ teaspoon
- Olive oil: 2 tablespoons

Directions:

1. Preheat your oven to almost 450°F. Set oven rack to the middle position.

2. Take one large bowl and combine rosemary, garlic, bread crumbs, pepper (1/4 teaspoon) and salt (1 teaspoon). Mix in olive oil (2 tablespoons) to moisten blend. Keep it aside.

3. Season the lamb rack with pepper and salt. Heat olive oil (2 tablespoons) in a heavy skillet over high flame. Sear lamb rack for almost 1 – 2 minutes on every side. Keep it aside for almost few minutes. Brush lamb rack with some mustard. Roll in the blend of bread crumbs to equally coat meat. Cover the corners of bones with a foil to avoid charring.

4. Arrange lamb rack (put rack bone area down) in a skillet. Roast lamb in a preheated oven for almost 12 – 18 minutes, based on your desire of doneness. You can adjust the cooking time as per your taste. Serve hot.

Recipe 67: Fish Fillets

Servings: 2

Cooking Time: 20 minutes

Ingredients:

- Cod Fish (2 fillets): 4 ounce
- Pepper and salt as per taste
- Greek Yogurt: 100 g
- Cooking Spray: Vegetable oil as per need

Directions:

1. Preheat an oven to almost 350F.

2. Sprinkle pepper and salt on the both sides of fish fillets. Put these fillets in one shallow oven-proof dish and spread yogurt over fish fillets.

3. Put this dish on the middle rack of your preheated oven and roast for almost 15 minutes until the yogurt starts bubbling and change its color. Serve hot with your favorite sauce.

4. If you want to cook on stove top, grease your cooking pan and put fish fillets. Cover this pan and cook for five minutes. Delicious fish is ready.

Recipe 68: Chickpea Salad

Cooking Time: 1 hour 5 minutes

Servings: 4

Ingredients:

- Chickpeas or garbanzo beans: 15 ounce
- Cucumber (finely chopped): 1
- Grape tomatoes (halved): 1 cup
- Chopped onion: 1/4 cup
- Minced garlic: 1 tablespoon
- Parsley flakes: 1/2 teaspoon
- Dried basil: 1/4 teaspoon
- Parmesan cheese (grated): 1 tablespoon
- Olive oil: 1 tablespoon
- Balsamic vinegar: 3 tablespoons
- Salt: 1/4 teaspoon
- Black pepper: as per taste

Directions:

1. Take a bowl and mix in cucumber, tomatoes, garlic, chickpeas, onion, parsley flakes, Parmesan cheese and dry basil.

2. Mix them well and drizzle with vinegar and olive oil. Sprinkle salt and pepper on these ingredients and toss them again.

3. Adjust seasoning as per your taste and cover this bowl to keep in your refrigerator for almost 45 minutes. Serve chilled.

Recipe 69: Tortilla Chips

Cooking Time: 25 minutes

Servings: 6

Ingredients:

- Corn tortillas: 12 ounces
- Ground cumin: 1 teaspoon
- Chili powder: 1 teaspoon
- Salt: 1 teaspoon
- Lime juice: 3 tablespoons
- Vegetable oil: 1 tablespoon

Directions:

1. Preheat your oven to almost 350F.

2. Cut every tortilla to make small wedges and arrange these wedges in one layer on your greased cooking sheet. Keep them aside.

3. Mix lime juice and oil in one mister and mix them well. Spray every tortilla wedge with this spray to moist them.

4. Take a bowl and mix chili powder, salt and cumin in this bowl. Sprinkle this mixture on the chips. Bake for almost seven minutes in a preheated oven. Rotate this pan and bake for 8 minutes again to make chips crispy. Serve with garnishes or salsa.

Recipe 70: Zucchini Chips

Cooking Time: 30 minutes

Servings: 2

Ingredients:

- Thinly sliced Zucchini: 1
- Pink salt as per taste
- Olive oil with garlic flavor: 1 tablespoon

Directions:

1. Preheat your oven to almost 375F.

2. Put zucchini slices in one bowl and drizzle ginger flavored olive oil over zucchini. Toss them well and sprinkle salt.

3. Spread these zucchini slices on a greased baking sheet. Bake in your preheated oven for almost 20 minutes. Serve with tomato sauce.

Recipe 71: Dinner Meatballs

Total Time: 1 hour 20 minutes

Servings: 8

Ingredients:

- Ground beef: 2 pounds
- Salt: ½ teaspoons
- Eggs: 2
- Chopped onion: ¼ cup
- Milk: ½ cup
- Barbecue sauce: 18 ounces
- Bread crumbs: 1 ½ cups

Directions:

1. Preheat oven to almost 375°F.

2. Combine eggs, salt, milk, onion, bread, and beef in one bowl and shape little meatballs (1-inch). Put meatballs into your greased baking dish and bake for almost 25 – 30 minutes.

3. Pour barbecue sauce over meatballs and bake for 35 minutes again. Serve over warm spaghetti.

Recipe 72: Salmon Cake

Total Time: 30 minutes

Servings: 4

Ingredients:

- Salmon (flaked and drained): 14.75 ounces
- Black pepper (ground): 1 teaspoon
- Whisked eggs: 2
- Vegetable oil: 3 tablespoons
- Diced onion: 1 small

Directions:

1. Remove all bones of salmon and separate all meat. Keep it aside.
2. Take one mixing bowl and whisk eggs in this bowl. Add pepper, salmon and diced onion in the bowl. Mix well.
3. Shape in two ounce patties (make almost 7 – 8 patties. Put one large skillet over medium flame and heat some oil. Fry every patty for almost 5 minutes on every side to make them golden brown and crispy.

Recipe 73: Chicken with Coconut Milk

Total Time: 30 minutes

Servings: 4

Ingredients:

- Ground cumin: 1 teaspoon
- Chopped onion: 1
- Minced ginger: 1 tablespoon
- Cayenne pepper (ground): 1 teaspoon
- Chopped and seeded jalapeno peppers: 2
- Ground turmeric: 1 teaspoon
- Minced garlic: 2 cloves
- Ground coriander: 1 teaspoon
- Chopped and seeded tomatoes: 3
- Boneless and skinless chicken: 4 breast (halves)
- Coconut milk: 14 ounces
- Pepper and salt: as per taste
- Chopped parsley: 1 bunch
- Olive oil: 2 tablespoons

Directions:

1. Take one medium bowl and mix coriander, turmeric, cayenne pepper, and cumin in this bowl. Put chicken in the bowl and season with pepper and salt as per taste. Rub all sides of chicken with the spice blends.
2. Heat olive oil (1 tablespoon) in one skillet over medium flame. Put the chicken in skillet and cook every side for almost 10 – 15 minutes to make it light brown and clear all juices. Turn off heat and put it aside.
3. Add remaining oil in the pan and heat it. Add garlic, jalapeno peppers, ginger and onion in the pan and cook for 5 minutes to tender.
4. Stir in tomatoes and keep cooking for 5 – 8 minutes. Mix in coconut milk and serve it over cooked chicken. Garnish with some parsley.

Recipe 74: Spinach Soup

Total Time: 30 minutes

Servings: 8

Ingredients:

- Olive oil: 3 tablespoons
- Ground allspice: ¼ teaspoon
- Chopped onion: 1
- Ground nutmeg: ¼ teaspoon
- Peeled & diced potatoes: 2
- Chopped celery: 2 stalks
- Chopped zucchini: 4 cups
- Minced garlic: 4 cloves
- Vegetable stock: 6 cups
- Minced ginger root: 2 tablespoons
- Cayenne pepper: 1 pinch
- Turbinado sugar: 1 tablespoons
- Chopped spinach: 1 cup
- Sea salt: 2 teaspoons
- Minced bell pepper (red): ½
- Ground turmeric: ¼ teaspoon

Directions:

1. Heat oil in one large pot or skillet over medium flame. Stir in sugar, ginger, garlic, celery and onion and cook them for five minutes to tender onion. Season with nutmeg, allspice, turmeric, and salt.

2. Add in zucchini and potatoes and stir in vegetable stock. Let this mixture boil and decrease heat to almost low and simmer for ten minutes to tender potatoes.

3. Turn off heat and season soup with cayenne pepper. Now mix in spinach and use one hand blender to blend this mixture and make it smooth. Garnish with some red bell pepper and serve warm.

Recipe 75: Beef Soup

Cooking time: 30 minutes

Servings: 2 to 3 servings

Ingredients:

- Dashi stock – 1 cup
- Soy sauce – ¾ cup
- Mirin – ¾ cup
- White sugar – ¼ cup
- Shirataki noodles – 8 oz.
- Canola oil – 2 tbsp.
- Sirloin beef (sliced) – 1 pound
- Onion (sliced) – 1
- Canola oil – 1 tbsp.
- Celery (sliced) – 2 stalks
- Carrots (sliced) – 2
- Green onions (pieces) – 5
- Mushrooms (sliced) – 4
- Tofu (cubes) – 14 oz.

Directions:

1. Get a bowl and mix sugar, soy sauce, and mirin and dashi stock.
2. Take a pot and boil the noodles for 2 minutes. Make sure you keep a check on it and then take it off to rinse with cold water.
3. Now get a pan and heat it with adding canola oil in it. Cook the beef in it for about 10 minutes until it is soft and tender.
4. When the beef is cooked, add celery, mushrooms, carrot and onion in it. Stir it well so all mix well. Now add the green onions along with the noodles, tofu and dashi mixture.
5. Now when the entire mixture simmers, then serve it in a big bowl to enjoy it with your family!

Recipe 76: Gherkins Salad

Cooking Time: 25 minutes

Servings: 4

Ingredients:

- Eggs: 8
- Brown mustard: ¼ teaspoon
- Dry mustard: ¼ teaspoon
- Mayonnaise: ½ cup
- Black pepper (ground) and salt: as per taste
- Green onion (chopped): 2 tablespoons
- Chopped celery: 2 tablespoons
- Paprika: ¼ teaspoon
- Chopped gherkins: 1 tablespoon

Directions:

1. In the first step, put eggs in one saucepan (in one layer) and cover all eggs with cold water. Place this pan on medium heat to let this water boil and decrease flame to low.
2. Cook eggs at low temperature for almost ten minutes. Turn off heat and drain hot water. Leave these boiled eggs under a running stream of water for a few moments to let them cool. Shell and chop eggs.
3. Stir dry mustard, brown mustard, gherkins, celery, green onion, mayonnaise and chopped eggs in a big bowl. Sprinkle pepper, salt and paprika over eggs and serve with crackers or fill in hollow tomato to serve.

Recipe 77: Shrimp Harissa

Cooking Time: 20 minutes

Servings: 2

Ingredients

- Frozen Shrimp: 30 to 40
- Water: ½ cup
- Spice mix (Ras-el Hanout): 1 tablespoon
- Chopped yellow onion: 1/3 cup
- Minced Garlic: 1 tablespoon
- Sea Salt: ½ teaspoon
- Chopped parsley (fresh): 1 tablespoon
- Chopped cilantro (fresh): 1 tablespoon
- Harissa sauce: 7 oz.
- Olive oil: 2 tablespoons
- Couscous (Cooked): 2 cups

Directions:

1. Preheat one oven to almost 400°F.
2. Wash shrimps with fresh water and let them boil in a pot filled with water for approximately 7 minutes on medium heat. Drain water and let them cool. Remove all shells on shrimps.
3. Put cooked prawns in one tagine bowl and add water, onion, mixed spice, salt, garlic, cilantro and parsley in this bowl. Now pour simmer sauce over the top and drizzle with some olive oil. Mix them well.
4. Keep this bowl in oven for almost 20 minutes without covering this bowl and in the meantime, use a stovetop to cook your couscous.
5. Take out this bowl from oven and put a tagine lid (cone-shaped) over to cover. Steam it for almost 5 to 10 minutes. Serve couscous and shrimp on a dish.

Recipe 78: Onion Soup

Cooking time: 30 minutes

Servings: 4

Ingredients:

- Celery (chopped) – ½ stalk
- Onion (chopped) – 1
- Carrot (chopped) – ½
- Ginger (grated) – 1 tsp.
- Garlic (minced) – ½ tsp.
- Chicken stock – 2 tbsp.
- Bouillon beef granules - 3 tsp.
- Mushrooms (chopped) – 1 cup
- Water – 2 cups
- Baby mushrooms (sliced) – 1 cup
- Chives (chopped) – 1 tbsp.

Directions:

1. Get a pot and add the following ingredients to it such as onion, ginger, carrot, garlic, celery and mushrooms. Mix it well and then adds the chicken stock. Stir the entire mixture and let it cook for 5 minutes.

2. When it comes to a boil, then add the beef bouillon along with water in it. Now cover the lid and let it cook for 10 minutes.

3. Now place the remaining mushrooms on the bottom of a bowl and when the mixture of soup is ready, then pour it over in the bowl. It will mix all the ingredients along with the baby mushrooms.

4. Sprinkle the chives over the bowl and serve when ready!

Dessert Recipes

Recipe 79: Apple Cake

Cooking Time: 30 to 40 minutes

Servings: 12

Ingredients:

- Baking powder: 1 teaspoon
- Baking soda: 1 teaspoon
- Brown sugar or sugar substitute: ¾ cup
- Eggs: 2
- Vanilla extract: 1 teaspoon
- Ground cinnamon: ½ teaspoon
- Nutmeg (ground): ½ teaspoon
- Raisins: ½ cup
- Salt: ½ teaspoon
- All-purpose flour: 2 cups
- Unsweetened applesauce: 1 ½ cups

Directions:

1. Preheat an oven to almost 350 degrees F and grease one loaf pan with non-stick cooking spray. Keep it aside.
2. Sift baking powder, baking soda, cinnamon, salt, nutmeg, and flour together. Keep it aside.
3. Beat all eggs and mix in sugar, vanilla, and applesauce. Add a mixture of flour in the egg mixture and beat well to make them smooth. It is time to add raisins.
4. Pour this batter into greased loaf pan and bake in your preheated oven for almost one hour. Insert a toothpick in the middle, if it comes out clean, your cake is ready. Serve chilled.

Recipe 80: Diet Bites

Cooking Time: 2 hours 20 minutes

Servings: 30

Ingredients:

- Cream cheese (whipped): 12 ounces
- Splenda granular: 2 tablespoons
- Brewed coffee: ¼ cup
- Vanilla/chocolate extract: ½ teaspoon
- Cool whip (fat-free): 1 cup
- Miniature tart shells: 30
- Raspberries: 30

Directions:

1. Take a bowl and combine Splenda, cream cheese, chocolate/vanilla and coffee in this bowl. Mix them well to make a smooth mixture and cover this bowl for almost two hours. You can put it in your refrigerator.
2. Mix in cool whip into Splenda mixture and use one spoon or pastry bag to fill tart shells. Top with raspberries and serve.

Recipe 81: Sugar-free Pie

Cooking Time: 2 hours 10 minutes

Servings: 8

Ingredients:

- Cracker Crust: 9 inch
- Sugar-free pudding (vanilla or chocolate flavor): 1 ounce
- Cold milk: 1 cup
- Crushed pineapple: 8 ounces
- Whipped topping: 8 ounces
- Chopped pecans: 1 cup

Directions:

1. Take a medium bowl and whisk milk and pudding mix in this bowl.
2. Mix in pineapple, pecans, and whipped topping.
3. Pour this mixture into prepared crust and chill for two hours before serving.

Recipe 82: Pumpkin Pie

Cooking Time: 1 hour 10 minutes

Servings: 6

Ingredients:

- Pumpkin puree: 15 ounce
- Skim milk: ½ cup
- Pie spice (pumpkin flavor): 1 teaspoon
- Fat-free whipped topping: 8 ounce
- Sugar-free pudding mix (vanilla flavor): 1 ounce

Directions:

1. Take one bowl and add pudding mix, milk and pumpkin puree in this bowl. Mix them well and add pie spice in this mixture along with whipped topping (only half).
2. Pour this mixture into your pie plate and spread remaining topping on the top of this pie. Keep in freezer for one hour or more. Serve chilled!

Recipe 83: Almond Bars

Servings: 1 bar

Preparation Time: 30 minutes

Ingredients:

- Almonds: ¼ cup
- Cacao Nibs: ¼ cup
- Figs: 3
- Cacao Powder: 1 tablespoon
- Goji Berries: ¼ cup

Directions:

1. Add almonds in the short cup of blender to grind them with the help of pulsing techniques to get a chunky consistency.
2. Put crushed almonds in one bowl and scoop out the whole meat of rips figs and put in the bowl with almonds. Add in goji berries, cacao nibs, and cacao powder.
3. Mix all these ingredients well and take handfuls of this mixture and make a rectangular bar. You can wrap each bar in a wax paper. You can shape the mixture once again after wrapping it in the wax paper.

Recipe 84: Apple Sorbet

Cooking Time: 30 minutes

Cooling Time: 4 hours 5 minutes

Servings: 8

Ingredients

- Smith apples (cored and sliced): 1 ¼ pounds
- Lemon juice: squeeze 1 ½ lemons
- Honey: 1 tablespoon
- Water: 1 ½ cups
- Sugar: 1 ½ cups

Directions:

1. Take a plastic container or resealable bag made of plastic and mix apples with lemon juice (1/2 juice) and freeze it for one night for a few hours.
2. Take one small saucepan and bring sugar and water to boil on medium heat. Decrease heat and simmer for almost five minutes. Turn off heat and mix in honey. Let this mixture cool completely.
3. Put the apple in the blender and liquidize these apples with remaining lemon juice and sugar syrup. Blend this mixture to make it smooth. Apple peels will give a unique texture to your sorbet.
4. You can transfer this blend to your ice cream machine and freeze it as per directions. Leave sorbet out for almost ten minutes before serving.

Recipe 85: Choco Dates

Cooking Time: 30 minutes

Servings: 25

Ingredients

- Chopped chocolate: 8 ounces
- Medjool dates (pitted): 25
- Pecan halves: 25
- Shredded coconut (sweetened): 2 tablespoons

Directions:

1. Put chocolate in a plastic or glass bowl and heat in your microwave for almost two minutes and stir after every thirty seconds to make it smooth.
2. Line your baking sheet with one aluminum foil and stuff every date with a pecan half and put on the baking sheet.
3. Drizzle melted chocolate on dates and sprinkle coconut over dates. Put these dates in the freezer and freeze for almost one hour. Serve with additional nuts as per your taste.

Recipe 86: Macaroon

Servings: 18

Total Time: 30 minutes

Ingredients:

- Olive oil spray
- Flaked coconut (unsweetened): 2 1/2 cups
- Unbleached flour: 1 cup
- Cashews: 3/4 cup
- Water: 3/4 cup
- Raw sugar (Turbinado): 1/2 cup
- Salt: 1/2 teaspoon
- Almond extract: 1/2 teaspoon

Directions:

1. Preheat your oven to almost 350 °F. Grease baking sheet with your cooking spray.
2. Combine flour and coconut in one large bowl.
3. Use a blender to puree almond extract, salt, sugar, water and cashews. Stir cashew blend into coconut blend and mix them well.
4. Make 1-inch balls from coconut blend and make these balls flat. Arrange these balls on greased baking sheet.
5. Bake cookies in your preheated oven for almost 12 – 15 minutes to make edges golden.

Recipe 87: Pancake

Cooking Time: 20 minutes

Servings: 8

Ingredients:

- All-purpose flour: 1 ½ cups
- Milk: 1 ¼ cups
- Egg: 1
- Baking powder: 3 ½ teaspoons
- Salt: 1 teaspoon
- Butter (melted): 3 tablespoons
- White sugar: 1 tablespoon

Directions:

1. Take one large bowl and sift baking powder, sugar, salt and flour together. Mix them well and make one hole in the middle and pour milk, melted butter and egg in the middle.
2. Stir them well to make a smooth mixture. Grease one frying pan and heat on medium flame.
3. Pour ¼ cup of pancake batter into hot frying pan and cook for 1/2 minute or more to let it brown and flip it to another side. Let the both sides brown and serve with your favorite syrup.

Appetizer Recipe

Recipe 88: Almond and Chicken Snack

Cooking Time: 55 minutes

Servings: 4

Ingredients:

- Chicken thigh (without skin and bones): 500g
- Red onion (thick wedges): 3 medium
- Red potato (thick slices): 500g
- Red peppers (remove seeds and cut into slices): 2
- Garlic (chopped): 1 clove
- Ground cumin + fennel seeds + smoked paprika (slight crushed): 1 teaspoon each
- Olive oil: 3 tablespoons
- 1 lemon: zest + juice
- Blanched almond (chopped): 50g

Serving Ingredients:

- Greek yogurt: 170g
- Handful parsley

Directions:

1. Heat your oven to almost 400F. Put your potatoes, onions, pepper and chicken in one large bowl and sprinkle seasoning.
2. Take one bowl, mix spices, garlic, lemon zest, oil and lemon juice together in this bowl. Pour this mixture over chicken and potatoes and spread this blend on two baking trays.
3. It is time to roast them for almost 40 minutes and turn over these ingredients after 20 minutes to thoroughly cook chicken. You can add almonds in last eight minutes of cooking.
4. Serve them in bowls with one dollop of yogurt and chopped parsley.

Recipe 89: Salmon with Soya Beans

Cooking Time: 25 minutes

Servings: 2

Ingredients:

- Omega-3 Egg: 1
- Soy beans (defrosted): 200g
- Lemon juice and zest: 1 lemon
- Oil (Flax seed): 2 tablespoons
- Puy lentils: 250g
- Spring onions (sliced): small bunch
- Salmon fillets (remove skin): 2 poached

Directions:

1. Put egg in one pan and cover it with chilled water. Let it boil on medium heat and cook for almost four to eight minutes. In the final minute, you have to add soya beans to this pan and drain. Run under fresh water and keep it aside. Remove shell of eggs and cut them into six wedges. Keep eggs and beans aside.
2. You have to mix the lemon zest and juice in a bowl with oil and seasoning. You can mix this blend in lentils, soya beans and onions in one bowl.
3. Divide this mixture between two plates and slowly break salmon in large pieces and put over lentils along eggs. You can enjoy it with brown bread.

Recipe 90: Chicken Skewer

Cooking Time: 50 minutes

Servings: 8

Ingredients:

- New potatoes: 500g
- Chopped parsley + chives + mint: 3 tablespoons each
- Olive oil: 6 tablespoons
- Lemon juice: 2 tablespoons
- Chicken breasts (without skin) 3cm chunks: 500g
- Red onion (peeled): 1
- Red pepper (remove seeds and 3cm chunks): 1
- Lemon (8 wedges): 1

Relish Ingredients

- Ripe Tomatoes: 8
- Green chilies (remove seeds and chopped): 2
- Garlic (chopped): 2 cloves
- Olive oil: 4 tablespoons
- White vinegar: 2 tablespoons

Directions:

1. If you want to use bamboo or wooden skewers, you have to soak them in cold water for almost half hour.
2. Boil potatoes in salted water for almost 10 to 12 minutes and drain. Put them aside to let them cool.
3. Take a mixing bowl and mix lemon juice, herbs, salt, pepper and oil in this bowl. You have to add potatoes and chicken in lemon juice mixture.
4. Mix them well to glisten everything. You have to cut onion to make six wedges and separate layers of each wedge. Add pepper and onion to marinate and mix them thoroughly.
5. Relish
6. For relish, you have to cut tomatoes and remove seeds. Chop them finely and mix garlic, tomatoes, oil, chilies, pepper and salt in tomatoes. Spoon this mixture into a dish.

7. Thread potatoes, chicken, onion, and pepper on eight skewers. Finish each skewer with one lemon wedge.
8. You can barbecue them directly on medium heat for almost 5 to 6 minutes on every side. You can serve with tomato relish.

Recipe 91: Lentil Sandwich

Cooking Time: 30 minutes

Servings: 4

Ingredients:

- Olive oil: 1 tablespoon + 2 teaspoons
- Red onion (diced): 1/4 cup
- Cooked quinoa (cook as per package instructions): 1 cup
- Brown lentils (drained and cooked): 1 cup
- Green chilies (diced): 4 ounce
- Rolled oats: 1/3 cup
- Whole-wheat Flour: 1/4 cup
- Cornstarch: 2 teaspoons
- Whole-wheat bread crumbs: 1/4 cup
- Garlic powder: 1/4 teaspoon
- Cumin: 1/2 teaspoon
- Paprika: 1 teaspoon
- Pepper and salt to taste

Honey Mustard Ingredients

- Dijon Mustard: 2 tablespoons
- Honey: 3 teaspoons

Directions:

1. Deep-fry onion in two teaspoons oil for almost four minutes on low heat.
2. Combine both ingredients of honey mustard and refrigerate honey mustard until you are ready to utilize it.
3. Combine all ingredients of burger in one mixing bowl and make four burger patties. In one large skillet, you have to add olive oil (1 tablespoon) in the pan and add patties to cook their both sides to let them brown. It will take almost 10 to 12 minutes. Enjoy these patties with your favorite roll or bun and spread honey mustard as your desire.
4. You can use sautéed tomato, romaine lettuce, tomato, mushrooms, honey mustard and mushrooms as toppings.

Recipe 92: Cornflakes Cookies

Servings: 24

Total Time: 30 minutes

Ingredients:

- Brown sugar (packed): 1 cup
- Diet sugar: 1/2 cup
- Softened butter: 1/2 cup
- Vanilla extract: 1 teaspoon
- Eggs: 2
- All-purpose flour: 3/4 cup
- Cornflakes cereal: 5 cups
- Flaked coconut: 1 1/2 cups

Directions:

1. Preheat your oven to almost 375 °F. Line your cookie sheets with dual parchment paper.
2. Cream white sugars, brown sugar, and butter in a bowl and add vanilla and eggs in this mixture. Whisk well.
3. Stir in flour and mix well to combine. Mix in coconut and corn flakes. Blend this mixture well and drop on a baking sheet lined with parchment paper by teaspoons.
4. Bake in your preheated oven for almost 8 – 10 minutes.

Recipe 93: Coconut Cookies

Servings: 8

Total Time: 30 minutes

Ingredients:

- Egg whites: 2 large
- White sugar: 1/2 cup
- Salt: 1/8 teaspoon
- Lime juice: 1 teaspoon
- Toasted and flake coconut: 7 ounces
- Cocoa powder (unsweetened): 1 tablespoon

Directions:

1. Preheat your oven to almost 300 °F. Line your cookie sheets with dual parchment paper.
2. Whisk egg whites until foamy in on metal or glass mixing bowl. Slowly add sugar and continue whisking to make soft peaks.
3. Now lift your beater or beat straight up. Egg whites may make soft mounds instead of sharp peaks. Add lime juice and salt and continue whisking until you notice a sharp peak that manages its shape as you stop whisking. Gently mix the cocoa powder and coconut in this mixture.
4. Drop this mixture via tablespoons on lined baking sheets. Bake for almost 20 minutes to make this mixture golden brown. Cool on pans and transfer to your wire racks. Store in one airtight container for later use.

Recipe 94: Chocolate Rice Bars

Servings: 24

Total Time: 1 hour 10 minutes

Ingredients:

- Butter: 1/4 cup
- Marshmallows: 10 ounces
- Chocolate flavored rice cereal (crispy): 5 cups
- Flaked coconut (Sweetened): 1/3 cup

Directions:

1. Grease a pan (9x13-inch). Take a large saucepan to melt butter over medium heat. Add all marshmallows and mix until dissolved. Turn off heat.
2. Quickly mix marshmallow blend into coconut and cereal to coat. Press in the greased pan with a buttered spoon.
3. Let it complete cool and cut into squares.

Recipe 95: Peanut Choco Bars

Servings: 24

Total Time: 40 minutes

Ingredients:

- Rice cereal (crisp): 8 cups
- Corn syrup: 1 cup
- Chocolate chips (semisweet): 1 cup
- White sugar: 1 cup
- Peanut butter: 1 ½ cups

Directions:

1. Butter a pan (9x13-inch).
2. Pour peanut butter, syrup and sugar in a microwave bowl. Put it in the microwave for 2 to 3 minutes on high, until it starts to bubble.
3. Once the mixture starts boiling, take it out from your microwave. Mix in chocolate chips and cereal until coated.
4. Pour this blend into greased pan.
5. Damp hands and sling off extra water. Press down blend into the greased pan and keep it aside to let it completely cool.
6. Cut it into squares.

Recipe 96: Baked Marshmallow Treats

Servings: 12

Total Time: 20 minutes

Ingredients:

- Butter-flavored cereal: 2 cups
- Butter (divided): ½ cup
- Breakfast cereal (fruity flavor): 2 cups
- Miniature marshmallows: 10.5 ounces
- Rice cereal (crispy): 2 cups

Directions:

1. Evenly grease butter in a baking dish (13x9-inch).
2. Put remaining butter in a non-stick pan over medium flame. Once melted, add marshmallow in melted butter and frequently stir for almost 5 – 7 minutes to complete melt marshmallow. Turn off heat.
3. Mix in crispy cereal, butter-flavored cereal, and brown sugar along with fruity breakfast cereal to coat all ingredients with marshmallow blend.
4. Pour this blend into a greased baking dish and press with the back of a spatula to flatten the mixture.
5. Let it completely cool before cutting its 3-inch squares.

Recipe 97: Choco Log

Servings: 12

Total Time: 1 hour 20 minutes

Ingredients:

- Large marshmallows: 10 ounces
- Crispy rice cereal: 5 ½ cups
- Chocolate chips (semi-sweet): 1 1/3 cups
- Butter: ¼ cup
- Butterscotch chips: ¾ cup
- Peanut butter: ¼ cup

Directions:

1. Line a pan (15x10-inch) with waxed paper. Grease this paper.
2. Combine peanut butter, butter, and marshmallows in a microwave-safe bowl. Cover this bowl and put in the microwave for almost 2 minutes over high to melt marshmallows. Stir well.
3. Mix rice cereal in marshmallow blend to coat well and spread on the greased pan.
4. Combine butterscotch chips and chocolate chips in your microwave-safe bowl. Heat this blend in your microwave for 2 minutes until melted. Mix well.
5. Carefully spread chocolate blend over cereal blend while leaving 1-inch boundary around edges. Roll cereal blend around sweet chocolate filling (jelly-roll style). Start rolling with its short side.
6. Slowly peel waxed paper while rolling and put the roll on a serving plate. Make sure to keep seam-side down. Set in the fridge for 1 hour. Cut into small slices.

Recipe 98: Crispy Rice Treats with Nuts

Servings: 12

Total Time: 1 hour 15 minutes

Ingredients:

- Almond butter: 1 cup
- Corn syrup: 1 cup
- Rice cereal (crispy): 6 cups
- White sugar: 1 cup
- Chocolate chips (dark): 2 cups
- Chopped almonds or nuts: 1 cup

Directions:

1. Mix sugar and corn syrup in a pan over medium flame for almost 5 minutes. Turn off heat and mix in almond butter and chocolate chips until melted.
2. Put rice cereal and ½ cup chopped almonds in a bowl. Stir in the almond-chocolate blend.
3. Pour this cereal into a baking dish (9x13-inch) and sprinkle with remaining chopped almonds. Cool for almost 1 hour before serving.

Recipe 99: Caramel Cheese Bars

Servings: 24

Total Time: 57 minutes

Ingredients:

- Caramel dip: 1 cup
- Cream cheese: 16 ounces
- All-purpose flour: 1 tablespoon
- Egg: 1 large
- Vanilla extract (pure): 1 teaspoon
- Cored and peeled apples (Granny smith): 2 (chop into ¼-inch slices)

Crust Ingredients:

- All-purpose flour: 1 cup
- Old-fashioned oats: ¾ cup
- Brown sugar: 1/3 cup
- Unsalted butter (chop into small pieces): 8 tablespoons

Directions:

1. Heat your oven to exactly 350°F. Grease a baking pan (9x13-inch).
2. To make a crust, combine all ingredients of crust in a bowl and mix well until crumbly. Press this blend on the base of the greased pan.
3. Bake for almost 10 to 12 minutes until light brown.
4. For filling, whisk cream cheese in a bowl to make it creamy.
5. Add caramel dip in the filling and mix it until smooth. Stir in vanilla, egg, and flour and mix well.
6. Pour cheese blend over hot crust and arrange slices of apple. Press them over cream cheese layer.
7. Bake for almost 20 to 25 minutes to let them cool to room temperature.
8. Cover this crust and chill in the fridge until firm. Spread caramel dip over bars before serving them.
9. Cut into small bars and serve. You can store leftover in your fridge.

Recipe 100: Brownie Bars

Servings: 24

Total Time: 45 minutes

Ingredients:

- Fudge brownies (traditional package): 19.5 ounces
- Egg: 1 large
- Vanilla extract: 1 teaspoon
- Chopped walnuts: ¾ cup
- Chocolate ice cream syrups: for topping
- Softened cream cheese: 16 ounces
- Condensed milk (sweetened): 14 ounces

Directions:

1. Set your oven to 350°F to preheat it.
2. Carefully prepare brownie mix after reading the instructions given on its package. Mix in nuts and spread this blend into a greased baking pan (13x9-inch).
3. Take a mixing bowl and whisk cream cheese in this bowl until fluffy. Slowly whisk in condensed milk, vanilla and egg until smooth.
4. Slowly pour this blend equally over brownie blend.
5. Bake it for almost 40 minutes in your preheated oven to make its top light brown. Let it cool and garnish with some chocolate syrup.
6. Cut into small bars and serve chilled. Store leftovers in the fridge, but choose a bowl with lid to secure them.

Conclusion

No doubt, with an endomorph diet plan, and exercise routine, you can avoid weight gain and lose weight. The diet plan requires you to avoid refined carbohydrates. Your body needs a mixture of healthy proteins, carbohydrates, and fats.

Make sure to consume nuts, vegetables, whole-grain foods, and fruits. For the best results, you have to do regular strength and cardiovascular exercises to boost metabolism, build lean muscles, and burn calories.

Decrease the consumption of refined carbohydrates and follow a workout plan. You have to follow a regular physical activity and portion control. With these healthy behaviors, you can shed extra pounds. It is essential to stick with a routine to shed extra pounds.

Made in the USA
Monee, IL
25 January 2021